WORKING IN THE KILLING FIELDS

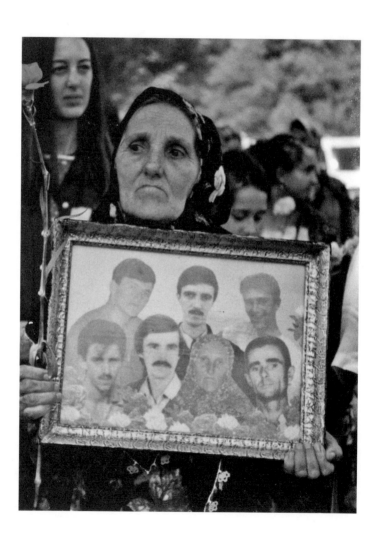

Working in the Killing Fields

Killing Fields

FORENSIC

SCIENCE

IN BOSNIA

HOWARD BALL

Potomac Books

An imprint of the
University of Nebraska Press

Portions of chapter 1 were originally published in "Incident at the Shore of the River Drina," Loquitor 18, no. 1 (Fall 2003): 14–18.

frontispiece: Muslim survivor holding a picture of missing family members. Bratunac, Bosnia and Herzegovina, 2003. Courtesy of the author.

Library of Congress Cataloging-in-Publication Data

Ball, Howard, 1937–
Working in the killing fields: forensic science in Bosnia / Howard Ball.
pages cm
Includes bibliographical references and index.
ISBN 978-1-61234-718-9 (cloth: alk. paper)
ISBN 978-1-61234-735-6 (epub)
ISBN 978-1-61234-736-3 (mobi)
ISBN 978-1-61234-730-1 (pdf)
1. Genocide—Bosnia and Hercegovina. 2. Yugoslav War, 1991–1995—Bosnia and Hercegovina. 3. Dead—Identification. 4. Disappeared persons—Bosnia and Hercegovina. 5. Forensic sciences—Bosnia and Hercegovina. 6. Bosnia and Hercegovina—History—1992–. Title.
DR1313.7.A85B354 2015
949.703—dc23
2014044972

Set in Scala by Lindsey Auten.

Dedicated to the Disappeared in War

"Sto te nema?" "Where Are You?" is the name of a Balkan folk song with roots going back many generations. The song is a mournful lament about a lost loved one and, understandably, became extremely popular during and after the Bosnian war. Its words captured the hearts of all the families—Bosniak, Croat, and Serb—about the thousands of disappeared during the war.

> When on a young field flowers
> Silent night collects pearls of dew
> A song comes flying through my heart
> Where are you, oh where are you?
> When the dream comes as comfort
> And soul prepares to rest
> From the heart the voice still asks
> Where are you, oh where are you?

CONTENTS

ACKNOWLEDGMENTS

There are dozens of residents and former residents of Bosnia and Herzegovina* I have met, there and in the United States, who have been of immense help to me in the writing of this book. Especially helpful have been Amor Masovic, presently one of the Directors of the Missing Persons Institute of Bosnia and Herzegovina, Sanela Basrambasic, who continues to work with the International Committee of the Red Cross, and Aida Sehovic, a former resident of Sarajevo, who came to the United States with her family and graduated from the University of Vermont in 1996. For many years, in America, Europe, and Sarajevo, she has presented her memorial to the disappeared annually on July 11, the anniversary of the Srebrenica massacre. It is called "sto te nema" and is in memory of the more than eight thousand missing Bosniaks.

There are a number of forensic scientists whose work in Bosnia and Herzegovina enabled me to understand the frustrations, the psychological stress, and the love they had for their work and the results of their successful identification of mortal remains on families of the missing. The writings of William Haglund, Eric Stover, Clea Koff, and Irfanka Pasagic, among others, gave me critical and revealing insights into the world of the forensic scientist.

*Throughout the book, Bosnia will be used in lieu of Bosnia-Herzegovina.

Their deep respect for the bones they found, cleaned, photographed, and identified left an enduring impact on my understanding of what they do and how they feel about their work. I hope I conveyed their humanity—a humanity that never left them—as they toiled endlessly in Bosnia's killing fields.

I was unable to return to Sarajevo and Srebrenica and therefore the Internet has been an invaluable source of information about events in Bosnia since my stay there in the spring of 2003. A number of sites gave me accurate and up-to-date information about the politics of the region and the efforts of courts—national and international—to bring the perpetrators of genocide and war crimes to justice. Some very helpful sites are Balkan Insight, Balkan Transitional Justice, and the Balkan Justice Report. Another set of valuable websites include those NGOs working to find and identify the disappeared, especially the International Committee of the Red Cross, the International Commission on Missing Persons, Amnesty International, Human Rights Watch, and Physicians for Human Rights.

Additionally, some UN websites were also very useful, especially the Human Rights Council, the High Commissioner for Human Rights, the International Criminal Tribunal for the former Yugoslavia sites, and the Working Group on Enforced or Involuntary Disappearances. I also thank the University of Vermont Retired Scholars Award Program for a timely grant supporting my research.

All of my sources, however, are not to blame for any mistakes in the book. I claim that responsibility. Finally, to Carol, the love of my life, thanks for always supporting my work for more than fifty years.

INTRODUCTION

On the Bank of the River Drina, May 10, 2003

Sixty-nine-year-old retired Yugoslav Army General Radko Mladic is presently before the International Criminal Tribunal for the former Yugoslavia (ICTY). He is charged under international law for the many orders he issued as military commander of all Bosnian Serb military forces between 1992 and 1995. The ICTY prosecutor's argument before the court is that these orders led to war crimes, crimes against humanity, and genocidal actions against Bosnian Muslim (Bosniaks) and Croatian civilians. He is being held in the International Criminal Court's prison in The Hague. His trial began in the summer of 2012 and continues in 2015.

On May 10th, 1992, based on one of Mladic's orders, Bosnian Serb paramilitary units swept into the Bosnian town of Bratunac, about 90 kilometers northeast of Sarajevo. The town was home for more than forty-five hundred Bosniaks and not too far from the town of Srebrenica where, in July 1995, a similar fate befell more than eight thousand Bosnian Muslim men—young and old—who lived or had sought protection in that UN-designated "safe haven."[1]

Like General Mladic, who was living freely in Serbia for more than a decade before his capture, many of those Bosnian Serb leaders who ordered the Bratunac, Sarajevo, and other genocidal actions are still at large and unpunished. Some, as Emir Suljagic noted in a *New York Times* op-ed piece, are still officers in the Bosnian Serb Army, and one is even a member of the Republika Srpska's (the Bosnian Serb entity created at the outset of the 1992–1995 Bosnian war) parliament.[2]

After crushing the armed resistance of the Bosniaks, the Bosnian Serbs continued their "ethnic cleansing" operation in Bratunac and surrounding Bosniak enclaves. The civil leaders—clergy, teachers, doctors, dentists, town clerks, and other civil servants—were immediately killed in gruesome ways. Typically, the Serb occupiers asked an ethnic Serb town resident to point out the important Bosniaks for execution. Peter Maass called the process "eliticide, the systematic killing of a community's political and economic leadership so that the community could not regenerate."[3]

After these executions, the women of Bratunac became separated from their brothers, fathers, husbands, and children and, after many were raped, were evacuated to the hamlet of Kladanj, more than fifteen kilometers distant.

The more than twenty-five hundred men and boys were taken to a school in town, Vuk Karadzic, and locked up. Over the next twenty-four hours, more than eighteen hundred Bosniaks died—slaughtered by the Bosnian Serb paramilitary groups. Their bodies were dragged and thrown into the nearby River Drina (which separates Serbia from Bosnia).

The remaining seven hundred Bosniaks, except for a few young men who escaped the massacre and who are witnesses to the Bratunac butchery, became new names in the International Committee of the Red Cross's Book of Missing Persons on the Territory of Bosnia and Herzegovina. This book, which has gone through many editions, maintains an up-to-date list of the names and last locations of the thousands of Bosniaks who "disappeared" during the 1992–1995 war.

The mothers, sisters, and wives of the dead and the "disappeared" relocated to Sarajevo and other Bosniak towns after the November 1995 Dayton (Ohio) Peace Accords ended the Bosnian wars. Joined by the women of Srebrenica and other Bosnian Muslim enclaves in the eastern part of Bosnia whose men disappeared, they created a nongovernmental organization (NGO) called the Movement Mothers of Srebrenica and Zepa Enclaves.

On May 10, 2000, the eighth anniversary of the massacre, the women took their first trip back to Bratunac, now in Bosnian Serb territory. They planned to visit the wooded slaughter area, walk to the River Drina, say prayers, and throw flowers into the river to honor their dead and their missing family members.

They did not reach their destination. On the outskirts of Bratunac, Bosnian Serbs who had moved into the homes and farms vacated by the Bosniaks were waiting for the four buses full of Muslim women from Sarajevo and from Tuzla. Although the vehicles were "protected" by Republika Srpska police and by NATO's Stabilization Force (SFOR) troops, they were unable to prevent the locals from throwing rocks, bricks, and other missiles at them. Windows on all four buses shattered; rocks and shards of window glass injured fourteen women. They received first aid but could not continue the trip. They returned to Sarajevo and Tuzla crestfallen.

I was visiting Srebrenica on May 10, 2003. I was in this part of the world as a Fulbright Distinguished Professor of International Law at Bulgaria's Sofia University College of Law—teaching a course entitled War Crimes and Justice. During the university's spring recess, I visited Bosnia, especially the two enclaves that had been the locales for crimes against humanity and genocidal actions by the Bosnian Serbs: Sarajevo and Srebrenica.

Accompanying me on the almost three-hour journey from Sarajevo to Srebrenica, located in once-hostile Republika Srpska, were my driver, thirty-one-year-old Adnan, a veteran of the wars who was seriously wounded four times, and my guide, twenty-seven-year-old Samira. Both are Bosniaks; both have felt the pain and terror, physical and psychological, of the three-year siege of Sarajevo. Both were reluctant to take me to Srebrenica but in the end they agreed to take me as long as I carried my U.S. passport.

Adnan borrowed a nondescript, beaten-up vw Golf auto from a friend of his because it is not wise to drive a new car through the Bosnian Serb countryside. For the entire journey to Srebrenica, a frightened Samira was crouched in the backseat for she did not want to see the Republika Srpska police—armed with machine guns—who dotted the roadside on the long drive to Srebrenica.

The visit to Srebrenica was a brief one, in part because there was not much to see other than the bullet-pockmarked houses, closed stores, and the few Bosnian Serb residents without jobs. It was also a brief stop because my two companions did not feel comfortable walking the nearly deserted streets of this once Bosniak-majority town. On the way out of town, we stopped at the memorial cemetery, still under construction, where some six hundred of the identified dead Bosniaks from the towns of Srebrenica and Potocari have been interred. We then decided to return to Sarajevo before it got dark.

At the town of Bratunac, a few kilometers from the cemetery, we came upon a small convoy of buses—escorted by more than one dozen NATO SFOR military vehicles. Police were lining the streets and were holding machine guns at the ready. We were informed by one of the policemen who held us up while the buses went through the town that the passengers were Bosniaks, mostly widows and orphans, coming from Sarajevo, about 80 kilometers distant.

Once again, this time eleven years after the massacre, these women were heading toward the Bosnia-Serbia border—the River Drina—and the last known site of the disappearance of their husbands, sons, and fathers. Impulsively, not until later aware of the tragedy that led these women back to this town and to the River Drina, we decided to follow the caravan.

We traveled another two or three kilometers before pulling off the road and getting out of the car. We were within a few meters from the River Drina. For a few moments, there were only the three of us, about two dozen Republika Srpska police—most smoking and some laughing—lounging around a deserted building (a former restaurant), a handful of news reporters, and a few well-dressed and suited civilians.

The buses had parked on the road, and we watched as nearly one hundred persons, mostly middle-aged and elderly women with a handful of teenaged boys accompanying them, slowly marched from the road to the bank of the River Drina. In the midst of the silent, solemn throng was a Muslim cleric. The marchers had red roses and other flowers in their hands as they made their way to the riverbank. Many women carried framed photographs of their missing family members.

They reached the bank of the River Drina and, after a brief prayer by the cleric and some of the women, the participants threw the flowers into the river to commemorate the eleventh anniversary of their dead and disappeared loved ones. They then gathered in small groups, said their own prayers, hands outstretched in worship, tearfully hugged each other, lingered a bit longer, and then slowly turned to march back to the buses for the long ride back to the security of the Muslim enclaves in and around Sarajevo. I glanced at the Bosnian Serb police, now Republika Srpska law enforcement people, and wondered how many of those men participated in the slaughter of the twenty-five hundred disappeared Bosnian Muslim grandfathers, fathers, husbands, sons, and boys eleven years earlier.

We drove back to Sarajevo without saying very much. The three of us, in different ways, were noticeably affected by the events at the riverbank.

The next week I found out more about the efforts of a few humanitarian agencies, governmental and nongovernmental, to help find the missing men and boys these women were mourning. In 1995 there were roughly 40,000 missing when the wars ended and 92 percent of them Bosniak civilians; most were male although there were also a small number of women and young girls. There is never an accurate count of the missing because of the tragedy that entire families are wiped out in the madness of all wars.[4]

The numbers of missing are not the extent of the Bosnian tragedy; they affect the lives of hundreds of thousands of others who still wait for them. The International Committee of the Red Cross (ICRC) calculated that, if there were about 40,000 missing in 1995, then 400,000 survivors were directly affected and, in 2015, many of them still lead a heartrending existence. "They are suffering a hell of a lot. It is a suffering different from others. It is the only suffering that gets worse with time."[5]

In 1993 Bosnian officials created a commission to assist surviving family members in locating their missing kinfolk. Staffed by less than two dozen men, all Bosniaks, their task was a gruesome one: locate the mass and individual gravesites (many victims were thrown into pits, some as deep as eighty meters), exhume the remains, try to identify the skeletons that were once Bosniaks, and determine how they died.

One major device, used by a small group of ICRC staff, is a "photo book" created to assist the survivors in identifying their missing family members. Like the Book of Names, this photo book has gone through many editions; it is now available for families to use in both entities: the Muslim-Croat Federation and the Republika Srpska.

The ICRC photo book is unusual for it contains photos of pieces of clothing and personal artifacts and accessories—bonnets, gloves, personal documents, sweaters, belts, wallets, shoes, socks—found on or near the skeletons of the thousands of bodies unearthed by the searchers of the disappeared. Typically, a family member of a missing person, with a psychologist sitting alongside, pores over these photos of bits of haberdashery in the melancholy effort to identify a loved one by the clothes—or eyeglasses, or wristwatch—the person wore at the time of disappearance.

I left Sarajevo that May of 2003 with a commitment I made to myself after seeing and speaking to the forensic specialists at work in the killing fields and in the morgues and small conference rooms in Bosnia. The tragedy of the disappeared and the activities of a handful of professionals are largely invisible to most people outside Bosnia. The task of locating gravesites, nearly all undisclosed, exhuming the bones, and identifying the dead goes on slowly, without fanfare and without sufficient human and financial resources to do the job more rapidly.

This grim activity goes on across the globe for sadly this onerous labor is the ubiquitous aftermath of war in our time. The principal focus of this book is to examine the work of these forensic professionals, the men and women who have committed themselves to the task of finding, exhuming, and identifying the disappeared in Bosnia.

ABBREVIATIONS

AAAS	American Association for the Advancement of Science, NGO
AI	Amnesty International, NGO
AMD	ante-mortem data
Bosniaks	Bosnian Muslims
CIA	Central Intelligence Agency (USA)
CIMIC	Civil and Military Cooperation (NATO)
DNA	deoxyribonucleic acid
EAAF	Argentine Forensic Anthropology Team, NGO
EU	European Union
EUFOR	European Union Force (in Bosnia)
FBiH	Federation of Bosnia (Bosnian Croats and Muslims), post-1995 entity (Dayton Peace Accords)
GFAT	Guatemalan Forensic Anthropology Foundation, NGO
HRW	Human Rights Watch, NGO
HVO	Army of the Bosnian Croats
ICC	International Criminal Court
ICJ	International Court of Justice
ICMP	International Commission on Missing Persons, NGO
ICRC	International Committee of the Red Cross, NGO

ICTY	International Criminal Tribunal for the former Yugoslavia (UN)
ICTR	International Criminal Tribunal for Rwanda (UN)
IFOR	Implementation Force (NATO) created under Dayton
IPTF	International Police Task Force (UN, ICTY)
IRCTV	International Rehabilitation Council for Torture Victims, NGO
JNA	Yugoslav Peoples Army (Serbian majority)
KFOR	Kosovo Implementation Force (NATO)
LMP	Law on Missing Persons (Bosnia)
NHS	National Health Service (Great Britain)
MPI	Missing Persons Institute (Bosnia)
MPID	Missing Persons Identification Resource Center (NGO)
NATO	North Atlantic Treaty Organization
NGO	nongovernmental organization
NLM	National Liberation Movement (Tito's Partisan Army)
NPA	Norwegian People's Aid (demining NGO)
OHCHR	Office of the High Commissioner for Human Rights (UN)
OSCE	Organization of Security and Cooperation in Europe
OTP	Office of the Prosecutor, ICTY and ICTR
PHR	Physicians for Human Rights, NGO
PMD	postmortem data
PROFOR	Protection Force (UN, after Dayton Peace Accords)
PTSD	post-traumatic stress disorder
RPG	rocket-propelled grenade
RS	Republika Srpska (Republic of the Serb People of Bosnia), post-1992 entity
RSOT	Operational Team of the Republika Srpska for Tracing Missing Persons

SFOR	Stabilization Force (NATO)
TRIAL	Track Impunity Always (NGO)
UN	United Nations
UNCHR	UN Commission for Human Rights
UNHCR	UN High Commissioner for Refugees
UNICEF	United Nations International Children's Emergency Fund (now: UN Children's Fund)
VMRO	Macedonian Revolutionary Organization
VRIC	Victim Recovery and Identification Commission (NGO)
VRS	Army of the Republika Srpska
WGEID	Working Group on Enforced or Involuntary Disappearances (UN, HRC)
WHO	World Health Organization (UN)

WORKING IN THE KILLING FIELDS

ONE

The "Disappeared" in War and the Need to Find and Identify Them

"The story of missing persons is not just a story about those who are missing, but a story about their families who remain, and wait."
—ANISA SUCESKA VEKIC

After an armistice or peace treaty ends armed conflict, there are many complicated problems that face the survivors, many of them refugees forced from their homes by an unsparing enemy.

One of the most pervasive tribulations facing the survivors is the agony of uncertainty regarding family members—both military and civilian—who "disappeared" during the hostilities. Where and what happened to the missing is a question inextricably linked to the political, legal, and psychological well-being of the surviving families. Are the missing noncombatants alive somewhere—in a prisoner-of-war camp, in a hospital, in another country—or are they dead, perhaps the victims of war crimes, crimes against humanity, or genocide.

If the missing loved one is alive, the family demands reunion so that some normalcy can return to their lives. If the disappeared is dead, the survivors want to know so that they can end the anguish of uncertainty. Finding an answer is vital to the social, physical, and mental health of the surviving family members.

In the last century, most of the civilians who disappeared in war or revolution were killed or murdered and closure is necessary. Religious reburial and legal closure (issuance of a death certificate) are two basic actions that can end the family's anguish.

Above all, however, there is always present the question of whether crimes against humanity, war crimes, and genocide occurred during the conflict, violating international laws of war. If the disappeared died because of criminal action, the perpetrators must face an accounting in a criminal court for their behavior during the conflict. Without justice, there is no solace for survivors and no lasting peace for the nation.

Indeed, the surviving family members continually demand information from oftentimes reluctant state authorities regarding the trial outcome of a perpetrator charged with committing war crimes that led to the disappearance of their loved ones.[1] Even the names of the indicted and those who were found guilty and sentenced to prison terms were, until recently, withheld from Bosnian families.[2]

Finding the Disappeared after Armed Conflict Ends

The *disappeared* is a worldwide heartbreak. In 1981 a coalition of Latin American and South American humanitarian NGOs established the International Day of the Disappeared, observed every August 30. It was launched in Costa Rica by citizens who wanted to keep the pressure on governments to find their disappeared after hostilities end. (The United Nations General Assembly officially recognized the day in 2010.)

The event is a sad but realistic acknowledgment of the harsh reality for hundreds of thousands of families who have relatives unaccounted for—many for decades—because of armed conflict. The ICRC is presently working with national organizations in more than forty nations on all continents to find the disappeared. In Africa, Asia and the Pacific, Europe, the Americas, and in the Middle East and North Africa, there are hundreds of international forensic specialists continually working to find, identify, and determine the cause of death of the victims.[3]

Some of the most controversial and still unresolved searches, going back to the 1950s, are in Argentina (1976–83, 13,000–30,000 missing), Bosnia and Herzegovina (1992–95, 40,000 missing), Cambodia (1975–79, 1.7 million killed, most disappeared), North and South Korea (1950–53, 87,000 South Koreans taken by North Korea), Iraq (1980–2000, 375,000–1 million [Anfal, Shi'ites, Marsh Arabs]; 2003–15,000), and Cyprus (1963–64, 1974, 2,000 still missing).[4] In some postwar countries, searchers cannot even begin the task of finding the disappeared. The new political leaders simply refuse to allow them into the former battle zones.

In every search by the ICRC and other governmental and nongovernmental organizations, there are four stages: (1) Searchers must find the disappeared. (2) They must identify the mortal remains so survivors can bury their long-lost dead. (3) There must be a forensic determination, if possible, of the cause of death. (4) The investigators must provide all recovered evidence to national and international criminal court prosecutors for determination of whether it substantiates survivors' accounts of war crimes, crimes against humanity, and/or genocide. If there are evidentiary facts, indictment and trial can follow after apprehension of the indicted persons.

The tragedy of the disappeared is a raw, emotional, and psychological one. It haunts the survivors, in many cases, throughout their lives. The wars in the former Yugoslavia from 1991 to 1995 were the bloodiest European events since the end of World War II in 1945.

The "Disappeared" in the Two Wars in the Former Yugoslavia, 1991–1995

In a 2011 report, the Demographic Unit of the Office of Prosecutor at the International Criminal Tribunal for the Former Yugoslavia (ICTY) published its research on the second Bosnian war.[5] Between 1992 and 1995, there was a mass exodus of more than one million refugees and internally displaced civilians and the deaths of *at least* 104,732 people.[6]

The vast majority of the victims of the first European genocide since 1945 were civilians of Muslim origin. Further, the number of persons still missing due to the war, in 1997, stood at 25,000.[7] "If one views this figure in the context of some 50,000 cases of disappearances in more than sixty countries in different parts of the world,[8] the number of cases of missing persons registered and unclarified in the former Yugoslavia is among the highest in the world."[9] In addition, in 2011, while the number of disappeared hovered around 30,000, "the *whereabouts* of between 10,000 and 11,500 people remain unknown."[10] The graves of one-third of the Bosnian missing are still undiscovered in 2015, two decades after the war ended. It grows more difficult to find and then identify the missing as time goes by.

The Impact of the Missing on the Family

The widow of a Croatian judge who disappeared when the Serbs attacked Croatians in 1991 said: "There is no greater suffering than not knowing where a loved one is buried."[11] Courtney Angela Brkic, a young forensic anthropologist and author, wrote poignantly about the tragic dilemma faced by these families of the disappeared: "There is a common denominator in refugee populations worldwide. . . . In the ranks of exile, there are women who listen each evening for a telltale sound coming from the hall outside their drafty rooms that says their husbands and children have returned, Lazarus-like. These women wait first one year, then another. They grow old in their waiting, each year like a ball of noxious mercury that combines with another, so that the passage of time is fluid and indistinct. They reject conflicting reports of massacres and the conventional wisdom that all is lost."[12]

Sanela Halilovic is the young wife of her missing Bosniak husband. Her haunting words echo the feelings of thousands of other women whose husbands still remain missing since the Bosnian wars ended in 1995: "Sometimes I tell myself that I would like to just know the truth about Mohamed because not knowing is killing me. But I do not want to know, because it's better to live with some hope, even a little. If I knew he was still alive, even if I knew I wouldn't see him for twenty years, I would somehow wait it out."[13]

A Bosnian psychoanalyst, Dr. Irfanka Pasagic, has written that for most survivors, "continuation of life means nothing more than a continuation of their suffering. Nightmares and flashbacks, thoughts and feelings as symptoms of the post-traumatic stress disorder (PTSD) from which most of them suffer, constantly return them to the center of the hell they survived."[14] It is clear from a number of studies of families of the disappeared—in Bosnia, Guatemala, Rwanda, and elsewhere—that they suffer a "sustained shock [as a result of] the anguish and pain caused by a missing loved one."[15]

For these persons full of pain, the "biggest loss is the loss of a child. The process of grieving in such cases sometimes lasts for a lifetime."[16] A family member cannot *mourn* a missing person properly. The missing are in limbo, neither alive nor dead. One forensic scientist wrote that she "knew mothers of disappeared children who, after almost thirty years, are still hoping for their missing child to appear."[17]

This book could just as easily have been called "What happened to my father," or "What happened to my brother, or to my mother, or to my husband, or, to my uncle, or, to my nephew, or, to my grandfather." Further, as Pasagic's and Brkic's words poignantly underscore, the reality is that life *stops* in so many psychological, personal, and cultural ways until there is an answer to the query. The answer, ultimately, is that missing persons are either dead or they are alive. However, as the International Committee of the Red Cross (ICRC) has so often found, "nearly all of the missing are dead."[18]

This evocative plea to find the disappeared is a ubiquitous one heard by visitors to all nations that experienced internal insurgent violence or armed conflicts (with an ensuing occupation) between nation-states. In the age of total war, innocent civilians disappear and their families instantly confront practical, personal, material, and financial hardships along with the psychological post-traumatic stress disorder associated with the disappearance.

Since 1996 Dr. Pasagic has worked with families of the missing in her office in Tuzla. She has observed one basic yet paradoxical fact: "All they wanted was truth. They want to know exactly what has happened to their missing husbands, fathers, and sons. It consumes them night and day. *Until they know the truth, they will never be able to grieve properly.*"[19] (my emphasis)

Because most of the disappeared are men, young and old, the family breadwinner has disappeared. Women in most parts of the world, traditionally and culturally, are heads of households and caregivers to both the young and old in the family. They are not breadwinners. They do not have marketable skills that translate into money to pay the bills. Speaking about her Bosniak women patients, Pasagic observed, "the absence of their men is a profound problem for the women. Many of them come from very rural communities and have little or no education. In our more traditional Muslim families, women take care of the household and tend the fields, while their husbands, who are usually the principal wage earners, work for hire or at jobs in town."[20]

When both parents are missing, the oldest child, often not yet a teenager, is left with the burden of maintaining the family. It is a tale too often experienced across the globe.

Compounding this dilemma is the fact that the larger society, whether in Argentina, Chile, Bosnia, or Rwanda, does not have the funds to provide the assistance needed for these families to exist as they did before the war. Without the necessary funds to sustain the woman who is head of the family, homes are lost and families are displaced. "They have no house, and no land, no men folk or communities to give them support. Alone, they must care for their children, their elderly parents or parents-in-law, and, of course, themselves. . . . They must become the sole breadwinners, a particularly frightening prospect in a world that is completely alien to them," commented Pasagic.[21]

There are, in most societies that face this dilemma of the disappeared, no entitlements or supports. Even in those situations where organizations such as the ICRC operate to assist these families, that support is not sufficient.

Rejha, a despairing Srebrenica wife and mother of four children, whose husband, Ismet, disappeared in 1995, recently said: "[My] younger ones, they ask about their father nearly every day. Our boy even talks to Ismet's picture." She said that birthdays and holidays are not celebrated, "not while our husbands and sons are missing. It wouldn't be right."[22]

The healing process for these families, from grieving to mourning and beyond, cannot begin until the "what happened" question is answered. Until then, there is the mostly unreasonable hope—because of the harsh and brutal reality of "ethnic cleansing"—that the missing person will one day reenter their lives, and time and life can begin again for the newly reunited family. And so the families, said Rejha, "talk about our towns and villages almost all the time. We remember what it was like before the war and how nice it would be to go back home and live like normal people."[23]

Furthermore, the family grieves incompletely for a very long time (and these families do not forget about the disappeared family member—even after three or four decades). In May 2003 I was in Nicosia, Cyprus, where on July 20, 1974, tens of thousands of well-armed Turkish troops invaded Cyprus, quickly defeated the Greek Cypriot militia, and from that time to the present have occupied almost half of the island nation. Yet four decades later, the tens of thousands of Cypriots who were forced from their homes and businesses by the Turkish occupiers cannot discount their pain and cannot forget their missing family members, their husbands and their sons.[24]

I was in a small shop looking at some beautiful hand-crafted linen and noticed framed photographs on an overhead ledge. I asked the shopkeeper, a delightful Greek Cypriot woman in her early sixties, about them. She instantly started to cry unashamedly. "They are photos of my husband, my two sons, and my nephew—all of them missing since the 1974 invasion." Evidently, her family lived in the area seized by the Turkish armed forces. The Turks let the women leave for the Greek Cypriot boundary but detained the male civilians. She has not seen them in almost forty years, but she still yearns for some closure before she dies.

Yet another dilemma for the survivors is confronting the reality that the perpetrators continually deny that genocide and war crimes took place. Ironically, "the fact is that both the victims and the perpetrators often want to forget what happened. The victim cannot do that regardless of how he or she tries, while the perpetrator is helped by the fact that the whole society wants to forget."[25]

"War and victims are something people would like to forget," wrote Judith Herman. "The veil of forgetting descends over everything painful and unpleasant."[26] Repeatedly, Bosniak survivors condemn the deniers (primarily ethnic Serbs) of the genocides and the ethnic cleansing. In 2005, a young forensic anthropologist working in the killing fields of Bosnia, herself a Bosniak, complained bitterly about what she termed "The Wages of Denial": "Ten years ago this week, Serbian forces slaughtered more than 7,000 Muslim men in the eastern Bosnian town of Srebrenica. Despite the efforts of a dedicated few in Serbia, and despite the war crimes prosecutions at The Hague, Serbia is no closer today than it was a decade ago to reckoning with its war guilt. For years, [Serbia] has denied involvement by its citizens in Srebrenica and other massacres of the 1990s."[27]

This reality for the surviving families, their inability to forget and the perpetrator's denial of the genocide, leads to stress-related psychological disorders, especially in the younger family members (the children of the missing fathers, mothers, husbands, and grandfathers). These mental problems affect all, from the wife (widow?) of the missing husband to the parents of that man, to his children. One particularly sad story shows in microcosm the nature of psychological trauma that occurs in a great many families of the disappeared.

Psychologist Pasagic told a journalist of a woman who had lost her husband and her five sons. She was forced to move away from her once-peaceful Muslim enclave in eastern Bosnia. She moved to a collective center for Bosniak families with her five daughters-in-law and several grandchildren. The oldest grandchild, a twelve-year-old boy, visited Pasagic's clinic because he had developed epileptic-like seizures. "Interviewing the boy," she noted afterward, "I discovered that he felt overwhelmed by the enormous expectations the women had placed on him to take care of the family. It was as if he had created his seizures as a way of crying out: 'Stop, I'm only a boy. I can't take care of all of you.'"[28]

The families of the disappeared are in a perpetual state of despondency. They spend their time trying to find out where their loved one is and what happened to him, and demanding revenge when they discover that their loved one was executed during an "ethnic cleansing" action. It is a "living" understood only by those who have been condemned, through the terrible fortunes of war, to live it.

A unique problem emerged once the Bosnian state prosecutors and judiciary began, in the first decade of the twenty-first century, the process of indicting and then trying accused war criminals. Until recently, some judicial bodies in the two post-1995 Dayton Peace Accords Bosnian entities (the RS and the Bosnian Federation) "[did] not include the indictees' identity in indictments [as well as not including] data about persons who have been sentenced for war crimes."[29] There have been demands made by national and international nongovernmental organizations (NGOs)—Survivors from Mostar and Blagaj and the International Commission on Missing Persons—that the surviving families receive this information about the processing of war crimes in Bosnia. The UN's ICTY processing of criminal charges, however, does make public *all* information regarding identity of the indicted and names of all those convicted and sentenced to prison terms for war crimes and genocide.

Focusing on the Problem of the Disappeared

The world has largely ignored this tragic consequence of war and revolution. Fortunately, however, governmental and nongovernmental organizations (NGOs) have not forgotten.

THE "DISAPPEARED" IN WAR

Humanitarian organizations such as the ICRC, Human Rights Watch (HRW), Physicians for Human Rights (PHR), and Amnesty International (AI) are assisting victims of war in a number of ways. Since the early 1980s, a number of forensic NGOs (the first group formed in Argentina in 1984 after the collapse of the military dictatorship) have performed a complementary task in the humanitarian effort to help the survivors: *finding* and *identifying* the survivors' missing family members.[30] These forensic groups have searched the killing fields in dozens of countries, from Bosnia to Iraq, from Rwanda to Guatemala.[31]

The work of these humanitarian NGOs is unbelievably difficult, for they all face a harsh reality. Within months of the end of a brutal war—the ethnic cleansing in Bosnia or the machete genocide in Rwanda—the world forgets about the "disappeared" and their forlorn surviving families. While the political leaders decry the violence that occurred in these bloodied territories and intone the words "never again," a few months later these same statesmen and prime ministers conveniently forget or ignore the recent horrors —until the next bloody war begins with its ensuing war crimes, crimes against humanity, and genocidal acts.

After the Bosnian war ends, with its brutality and crimes against humanity caught by cameras and splashed on twenty-four-hour cable television newscasts in nearly two hundred nations, life continues again—except for the survivors of that war. After the peace accord, the nation changes dramatically. The society that the Bosniaks, Bosnian-Croats, and Bosnian Serbs called homeland has disappeared. Afterward, three psychologists wrote, "the society in which the survivors lived no longer exists. . . . Traumatic events dominate individual destiny to such a massive extent regarding the number of persons affected, the frequency, intensity and duration of the events, we can expect a form of collective traumatization."[32]

The survivors of the cruel war are left largely on their own to cope with their personal tragedies, ailments, and needs—medical, psychological, economic, housing, education, and food and shelter. Beyond coping with these dilemmas in a new and dysfunctional nation, there is, for thousands of families, the overriding crisis: where are the disappeared? Finding them and meting out justice to their executioners is "essential to reconciliation and peace," said former U.S. senator Robert Dole in 1997. He was the president of the newly created International Commission on Missing Persons (ICMP) and understood the importance of resolving the problem. "Identification," he said in Sarajevo, "can bring closure to thousands of families who have been locked into the torment of the past and unable to move towards the promise of the future."[33]

Two decades after the Bosnian war ended, there is still no closure for thousands of Bosnians. For the Bosniak survivors but also Croat and Serb survivors, there is no forgetting the disappeared. It is a "not-forgetting" that, for many, will last a lifetime. There is the reality of the community suffering from PTSD; although the nightmares and the insomnia and the other painful manifestations of this illness may moderate over time, they remain until the missing are found or the survivors die—whichever comes first.

Christina Navarette is a Chilean psychoanalyst who attended the 2001 Ernest Jones Lecture given by South African justice Richard Goldstone. She offered an important insight into that evening's topic, which was a talk by Goldstone, the first chief prosecutor of the ICTY, entitled "Crimes Against Humanity—Forgetting the Victims."[34]

Many persons, she observed remorsefully, are twice victimized by genocide. First, though scarred by the crimes against humanity and the genocidal actions they experienced, they have somehow survived the bloodbath. However, they become victims a second time because they have expectations about quick justice for them and their dead and/or missing family members that do not materialize. Repeatedly, the global community beyond their nation's borders has simply forgotten about them and about the immense value of justice's "healing balm."[35]

The survivors become victims a third time, however, because the world's forgetfulness has denied them the financial and professional assistance needed to find the missing and to identify as many of them as scientifically and humanly possible. Surely, this is an intolerable situation for the survivors.

"Victimhood" continues long after the bloodshed ends— for a lifetime in many instances. "The family structure under such circumstances is totally disturbed and has very significant negative circumstances, in particular for children."[36] For example, eight hundred thousand were massacred in Rwanda in three months in the spring of 1994; immediately afterward, in sixty thousand Rwandan homes, the oldest family member was less than sixteen years old, Justice Goldstone noted in his talk.

Psychologists the world over probably agree that there is an understandable dynamic to forgetting. To forget is to defend against pain, guilt, trauma, and helplessness. These, however, are precisely the attributes of "victimhood." The mothers, wives, and daughters of the disappeared are chronic sufferers of pain, and guilt, and trauma, and hopelessness. They cry themselves to sleep nightly; they really do not sleep because of their nightmares.

Clearly, financial assistance and professional expertise are needed to help these survivors cope with the punishing aftermath of the Bosnian war. Paralleling these human needs is the necessity of continuing efforts to find the disappeared and provide prosecutors at the ICTY and in the Bosnian criminal court system with the evidence necessary to prosecute the perpetrators of crimes against humanity and genocide. There must also be the appearance of more conscience-driven military veterans to inform the searchers of the missing about *where* the bodies can be found.

Ironically, the world's forgetfulness comes at a time in history when the numbers of civilian casualties in wartime have dramatically increased. In the twentieth century, war became total; the *entire* population of embattled states—combatants and civilians—felt the consequences during and after the battles. In 1900, data for casualties and the disappeared for nineteenth-century wars listed military combatants more than 90 percent of the time. A century and two world wars later, almost 80 percent of casualties and missing of *all* wars in the twentieth century were civilians. Bosnia's data underscores the flip-flop of this data: more than 90 percent of the disappeared are civilians, mostly men and boys, but including infants as well as elderly pensioners.

In the first two decades of the twenty-first century, more than fifty wars were raging around the world. In all these war zones, tens of thousands of families are trying to cope with the consequences of the absence of the family breadwinner, most of whom are civilians. Whether in Bosnia or Iraq or Sudan, survivors insistently demand that the missing be found and that perpetrators be caught and punished for their crimes against innocent noncombatants. The ICTY was an ad hoc criminal justice organ created by the UN in 1993 in response to intense media criticism of the UN's unwillingness to end the Balkan wars. The creation of the ICTY, and the ICTR one year later, were reactive responses by the UN to genocidal warfare in Bosnia and Rwanda. In both wars, there was no political will present to send UN military into these battlefields to end the horrors.

These tepid actions by the UN in response to the genocidal wars continued the drumbeat by a number of small concerned UN-member nations to establish a more significant, and permanent, international criminal justice system. This insistence, accompanied by the spectacle of regional bloody wars, led to a watershed event in Rome, Italy, in the summer of 1998. More than 160 of the then-185 member-nations of the UN (there were 193 members in 2015) participated in the Rome Conference on the creation of a permanent international criminal court. The conference, formally called the UN Diplomatic Conference of Plenipotentiaries on the Establishment of an International Criminal Court (ICC), ended on July 17, 1998. The conference required a two-thirds vote of the 161 UN-member nations (107) to pass the final draft of the treaty; 120 nations approved it. Only seven nations, the United States, China, Israel, Libya, Iraq, Qatar, and Yemen, voted against the treaty.[37] Under terms of the treaty, the ICC would come into being, as an independent, permanent organization, but not a part of the UN system, when ratified by sixty governments, who are members of the UN. The ICC came into force on July 1, 2002. It is based in The Hague, the Netherlands. It has *complementary jurisdiction* to hear cases involving war crimes, crimes against humanity, and genocide. Complementary jurisdiction can be applied by the ICC only if the nation state where the alleged violation occurred cannot or will not indict and try the perpetrators in its courts. A second (hoped-for) reason for the ICC is that its existence would deter future leaders bent on genocidal slaughter from acting on such inhuman impulses. Given the geopolitical realities inhabiting the international arena in the post–Cold War era, this new international court faces arch critics who believe that the ICC, with its limited jurisdiction to hear cases addressing controversial crimes, is incapable of dealing with these intense clashes with equanimity and punishing the guilty in a manner befitting the crimes they committed.[38]

In Bosnia, many survivors of the ethnic cleansing terrors have expressed grave reservations about the work of the ICTY (and, by implication, the ICC). They have repeatedly said that "European civility [evidenced by the working of the ICTY] is shit" because, to their eyes, the guilty evade *real* punishment in these trials. The death penalty is forbidden and so the planners and the implementers of the genocide live, unlike the death penalties meted out to convicted Nazis and Japanese by the Nuremburg and Tokyo war crimes tribunals. The ICTY's unfairness is enhanced by the very western-style plea-bargaining arrangement worked out by indicted military leaders and the ICTY prosecutors' office. As an example, the critics point to the pre-trial events involving Momir Nikolic, an officer in the Bosnian Serb military, and prosecutors. A deal was cut that enabled Nicolic, who was charged with genocide because of his participation in the slaughter of thousands of Bosniak civilians in Srebrenica in July 1995, to avoid a harsh sentence. He pled guilty to the charges but, because he testified as a witness for the prosecution against other Bosnian Serb military accused of the same crime, he received a twelve-year prison sentence.

This plea bargaining reality has led to a not-unexpected response by the survivors of these crimes: revenge. An angry male survivor of the Srebrenica genocide reflected the anger of his cohort when he said he could never return to his former home and live alongside Bosnian Serbs. He would seek revenge against the Serbs who killed his father and his brother if he met them.

Forensic Science Answers the Questions about the Missing

The only persons who have the capabilities, skills, and knowledge to find the disappeared, so that the wife of a missing spouse can say, finally, "Yes, I am a widow," are the world's forensic scientists, men and women committed to answering the questions surrounding the dilemma of the missing. While the ICRC and other NGOs inform the world about the tragedy and work with the families of the missing, it is the relatively small band of forensic scientists who handle the dirty work of finding, exhuming, and identifying the bones found in mass and individual graves in every nation that has experienced war or revolution.

After the graves are discovered, the forensic scientists extract DNA (a breakthrough first successfully implemented in 2001) from the bones and compare their findings with DNA samples collected, and placed in a computerized database, from tens of thousands of surviving family members. After they have identified the human remains using DNA, they share the information with the surviving family members as well as with investigators for war crimes tribunals—the ICTY and the Bosnian prosecutor's office—and, in the future, may do so with the newly created ICC in The Hague.

The prosecutor's task, following the bloodshed and the horrors of a war, is to indict and convict someone of a war crime or crime against humanity. To do this, the prosecutor must establish that a crime has been committed and whether that criminal activity is part of a state "policy of killing outside of combat. In a war crimes case, forensic anthropologists and pathologists have. . . . to prove that the killings were unlawful and not part of regular combat [which is the ubiquitous claim of the perpetrator]."[39]

Forensic science in the quest to dispel the lack of knowledge about death and murder in war zones is a relatively new field. Forensic science begins "when people die."[40] These professionals, using modern technology, must establish who the victims were and whether war crimes occurred in Bosnia, Rwanda, and other war venues. As Koff notes, the "mandate" of the forensics team "was really quite simple and straightforward":[41] finding mass grave sites, carefully uncovering them, exhuming the bodies, and analyzing the mortal remains and the evidence associated with the bones in order to establish whether or not crimes against humanity had been committed.

Often the evidence of murder was crystal clear. In many killing fields in Bosnia and elsewhere, forensic anthropologists "discovered wires that had been used to bind wrists on many of the bodies and cloths had been used to gag or blindfold people who had also been shot to death." "This kind of evidence," said a forensic anthropologist about her work in Bosnia, "corroborates witness testimony by survivors."

> We recovered bullets from the bodies, and bullets and shell casings around the gravesites because ballistic analysis can help establish which forces were doing the shooting and where the shooters were standing at the time. . . . We are always trying to understand the relationship between the bodies and the shooters: was the person who was shot facing the shooter, was the person made to get in a grave before they were shot. We collect this evidence to establish whether the people were combatants or civilians, whether they were prisoners of war who had surrendered, or if they were wounded when they were killed. . . . Each of these answers helps us to re-create these last moments.[42]

Working in Rwanda, Croatia, Bosnia, and too many other killing fields, the forensics experts uncovered remains that had two or three sets of clothing on them, or civilians murdered who had X-rays of their injuries hidden underneath their hospital garments. The dead evidently had prepared themselves for movement to another place or another hospital; "they expected to survive perhaps in another town, perhaps after returning from a refugee camp." They were not prepared to be executed by their captors.[43]

As will be seen in chapters 3 and 4, the term forensic science is a collective phrase, encapsulating a variety of forensic specialists from medicine and health care, science, and other technical professions. Forensic specialists from medicine and health care include forensic pathologists, forensic odontologists, and medical epidemiologists. Forensic specialists from the sciences include forensic anthropologists and osteologists (who specialize in bones), molecular biologists, botanists, archeologists, radiographers, ballistics experts, forensic entomologists, and firearms specialists. Finally, technical forensic specialists include evidence handlers, photographers, interviewers, police, ordnance experts, mortuary technicians, and administrators who manage the exhumation site and the morgues.

This book focuses on the emotional, legal, historical, political, and material questions associated with the work of forensic scientists:

(1) finding the "disappeared" in Bosnia

(2) identifying the mortal remains—and the cause of death—after the Bosnian war ended, with the help of newly developed protocols allowing forensic scientists to extract DNA samples from the bones of the dead[44]

(3) providing the evidence of murder and crimes against humanity to the ICTY prosecutors and other national criminal court personnel for use in criminal trials at The Hague and Bosnia. Finally

(4) informing the survivors of the news and providing them with the remains of their missing family member so that the dead can be properly interred. For Bosniaks, funerals and burials "are religious rites of passage for the survivors. [They] view bereavement as an experience to be shared, strengthening the solidarity of family and community. ". . . The absence of the bodies was robbing them not only of the rituals but of the visual cues that would help them to acknowledge the deaths of their loved ones and to pass through states of mourning and grief."[45]

The book's primary focus is the forensic scientists, the committed and courageous men and women who have worked in Bosnia since the mid-1990s in the often agonizingly slow, tedious, dangerous, and frustrating process of finding and then trying to identify the cadavers of those who disappeared during warfare. Many people have dedicated their lives to finding the missing.

My goal in chronicling the events depicted in the book is to place them in the public eye because they have gone about quietly tackling, head on, a human, medical, legal, and moral problem of the greatest magnitude. By their actions, these forensic professionals from across the globe have enabled prosecutors to indict and convict war criminals. Equally valuable, their findings have also brought some kind of closure to the families living in suspended animation pending information about their loved ones who "disappeared."

TWO

Balkan Nationalism, the Creation and the Collapse of Yugoslavia, and "Ethnic Cleansing"

The whole country is one huge mass grave—the place is a huge killing field.

—IRFANKA PASAGIC

The Yugoslav wars of the 1990s have reminded us of the lethality of Balkan nationalism.

—CHRISTOPHER CLARK

Throughout history, the Balkans, labeled by historians as the tinderbox of Europe, have been a crossroads whose troubles have ignited wider wars. It has been a zone of endless military, cultural, and economic mixing and clashing between Europe and Asia, Christianity and Islam, Catholicism and Orthodoxy. Moreover, for the past two centuries, Serbia has been at the center of many of these clashes.

When the 1992 Bosnia-Serbia war began, the Balkans was a region with "a political and cultural history unlike that of any other . . . in Europe." The great religions and political powers of Europe overlapped and combined there across the centuries, including "the empires of Rome, Charlemagne, the Ottomans, and the Austro-Hungarians, and the faiths of Western Christianity, Eastern Christianity, Judaism, and Islam."[1]

Both Serbs (in the thirteenth and fourteenth centuries)

and Croats (in the tenth and eleventh centuries) emerged as powerful medieval Slavic states. The Croats accepted Roman Catholicism and fell under the influence of the Vatican. In 1102, Croatia was conquered by Hungary and became a part of the (Roman Catholic–majority) Austro-Hungarian Empire until its defeat in World War I.

The Serbs became members of the Eastern Orthodox Church in the early decades of the fourteenth century. In 1389, however, Turkish forces defeated Serbian-Christian armies in the battle of Kosovo Field and began the Ottoman occupation of Serbia, which lost its independence in 1459.[2] By the middle of the fifteenth century, Ottoman forces controlled the Western Balkans—Serbia and Bosnia.

The "most distinctive and important feature of Bosnian history" under the Turks was the "Islamicization of the large part of the population after 1453."[3] The Muslim Slavs, over 150 years, grew quickly. In 1548 the Muslim population was 40 percent of the total; by the early seventeenth century, Muslims became an absolute majority in Bosnia.[4] During this time, even though it was not Ottoman policy to convert people to Islam, and Christians and Jews continued to practice their religions,[5] many thousands of Serbians moved out of the Ottoman Empire into areas controlled by the Austrian monarchy.[6] Given this reality, Croatia remained a Roman Catholic entity.

There is, however, a fundamental irony present in this region. Even though Croats (Catholic), Bosniaks (Muslim), and Serbs (Eastern Orthodox Christian) may worship God in different ways, they are all Slavs. They look like each other. They dress alike. Most speak the same language: Serbo-Croatian. Over the centuries, about 20 percent intermarried and, especially in Bosnia, the three Slavic peoples lived next to each other in all three countries. As a Serb living in Bosnia told a reporter at the beginning of the Balkan wars of the 1990s: "We all lived in Visegrad like a big family, the Muslims and the Serbs. Everyone had mixed marriages. We never tried to find out who was a Serb or a Muslim. We didn't look for differences. You know, it wasn't the people who wanted to fight. It was the politicians who prepared this stew, and now we can never go back."[7]

A journalist noted that "the truth of the matter is that *all* the combatants [in the Bosnian wars of the 1990s] were the same ethnic group—Slavic."[8] A young Serb living in the heavily Bosniak-populated town of Gorazde wrote that all his neighbors "had gone to the same schools, spoken the same language, and listened to the same music." Yet "overnight [they were] blinded by ethnic hatred and start[ed] to brutally kill one another."[9]

The Bosniaks lived largely in the cities, working in local government and the professions. Over the centuries of Turkish rule and afterward, the mostly non-practicing, liquor-drinking, pork-eating Muslims were Bosnia's elites. Serbs and Croats generally lived in the countryside and toiled as farmers. They were, one journalist wrote, "the country bumpkins."[10]

The Emergence of Serb Nationalism and the Vision of a "Greater Serbia"

The early Serb empire collapsed when defeated by the Turkish military on Kosovo Field in June 1389.[11] Ever since, the restoration of this medieval state has become "the expression of an ancient historical right."[12] This Serb vision has repeatedly led to wars, ethnic hatred, assassination of opposition leaders, and slaughter in the Balkans for more than six hundred years. "Wars," wrote Max Hastings, "seemed to work well for them."[13]

In 1844, a secret government document "became the Magna Carta of Serb nationalism."[14] Written by Serb interior minister Ilija Garasanin for Prince Alexandar Karadjordjevic, it has an inoffensive-sounding title: "A Program for the National and Foreign Policy of Serbia." Its central, unchanging first commandment accounts for the brutal history of the region since then: "*Where a Serb dwells, there is Serbia.*" This "expansionist vision of national unity," the unification of all Serbs within the to-be-created boundaries of a Greater Serbian state, became the "policy blueprint" for Serbian rulers. It explains Balkan history since then.[15]

Nationalist propaganda spread this pan-Serb vision to the population through patriotic press networks. It was, additionally, deeply embedded in the Serb "culture and identity" through the "extraordinarily vivid tradition of Serbian popular epic songs. These songs established a remarkably intimate linkage between poetry, history, and identity."[16]

Also at this time, the Eastern Orthodox Church became the religious apologist for this visionary Serb nationalism. "The Church [became] more of a nationalist than a religious organization. Serb priests mythologized the defeat of the [1389] battle of Kosovo and demanded that it be avenged."[17]

For nearly a century, Serb nationalists called for a continuous struggle against the infidel empires in order to create this Greater Serbia. However, their vision clashed with the ethnic reality that existed then and continues to exist today. The quixotic nationalistic paean ("Where a Serb dwells, there is Serbia") continually confronted the ethnic reality of the region: Serbs were not then—and not now—in the majority in Croatia, Bosnia, or Kosovo!

Nevertheless, Serbs acted on this fiction. There arose, in the late nineteenth and early twentieth centuries in Serbia, small terrorist groups such as the Serbian National Defense, the Union or Death (popularly known as the Black Hand), and the Independent Radicals. Their goal was to foment violent revolutionary action in these lands controlled by the alien empires in order to realize their vision of a Greater Serbia.

In their activities, the young nationalists received covert financial and technical support from the government in Belgrade. Much like contemporary terrorist groups such as the Irish Republican Army (IRA)[18] or Al Qaeda, these secret Serbian groups recruited young zealots who entered terrorist training camps, where they were instructed in marksmanship, bomb-making and -throwing, bridge-blowing, espionage, and political assassinations. They carried out violent acts in the effort to force the "infidel" regimes to exit these Balkan regions.

In 1908, the Dual Monarchy (Austria-Hungary), victorious over the Turkish army, formally annexed Bosnia. Serbian nationalists were apoplectic. This action "created an unparalleled outburst of resentment and national enthusiasm" in Serbia (and Russia[19]). Speakers at rallies across the nation called for war against the Austrian-Hungarian Empire. There was the uncontrolled clamor for an "armed crusade to retrieve the annexed provinces."[20] It was, realistically, a very dangerous strategy: there was no way Serbia's armed forces could hope to defeat the Hapsburg Empire's army.[21] Advised by the Russians, British, and French to desist in such a hopeless campaign, the Belgrade government formally renounced its demands on March 31, 1909.

Afterward "no responsible minister could afford openly to disavow the national program of Serbian unification."[22] These events led to the further radicalization of the Serbian revolutionary movement and to an unbridgeable chasm between the Belgrade government and the radical groups, who continued to plot secretly and to carry out acts of political terrorism, including assassinations in these conquered provinces. Ignored in all the shouts and cries for a war for the liberation of these annexed lands was the historic reality that they were never a part of the medieval Serbian empire of Tsar Dusan!

Between 1911 and 1914, there were nearly two dozen actions to murder "infidel" opponents of Pan-Serbism, capped off by the assassination of the heir-apparent to the Austrian-Hungarian throne in Sarajevo on June 28, 1914. A young Serb terrorist, Gavrilo Princip, a member of the Black Hand, killed the Hapsburg Monarchy's Archduke Franz Ferdinand and his wife Sophie, ushering in World War I a month later. Not only was the event committed on the royal couple's fourteenth wedding anniversary, but more important, "it was also a date pregnant with painful significance for Serbs"—it was the anniversary of the Serb defeat by the Ottomans in 1389.[23]

It was the beginning of a tumultuous global conflagration that, over four years, changed the world in fundamental ways.

An Impossibly Difficult-to-Govern State: Yugoslavia, 1918–1980

What we know as Yugoslavia came into existence in 1918 when, after the victorious allies divided up the defeated European powers' lands, taking territory away from the Germans, Turks, Austrians, and Hungarians, new nations and protectorates were created across the globe.[24]

In 1918, the newly created Slavic state, led by the Serbian monarch (Peter I, 1918–1921), was born. It stretched from the western Balkans to Central Europe. Called the Kingdom of Serbs, Croats, and Slovenes, it included the Austrian crown province of Bosnia, the former Austrian-Hungarian territories of Croatia and Slovenia, Macedonia, and the formerly independent Kingdom of Serbia-Montenegro. Eleven years later, in 1929, the nation officially became the Kingdom of Yugoslavia ("land of the south Slavs").

The specter of unvarnished nationalistic actions immediately emerged in the newly created Kingdom of Serbs, Croats, and Slovenes. Within a few years, "Serbian nationalism was [once again] the most disruptive force" in the Kingdom.[25] (Serbia was the only nation-state that was part of the "process of the formation of the [Kingdom]."[26])

The Interwar Years, 1918–1939

The Kingdom was created from a number of regions that, before the First World War, "belonged to different countries and underwent very different economic and cultural development. This resulted in very different political, cultural, and economic legacies and different regional and religious characteristics."[27] From its inception, there were disagreements between Serbian leaders who continued their quest for an enlarged, greater Serb nation and Croat and Slovene politicians of the new Kingdom who wanted a viable unified nation.

In 1920 the initial elections in the Kingdom reflected this division. Votes, cast along ethnic and regional lines, led to unstable coalition governments, a weak parliament, and an increasingly strong monarchy. After the 1921 Constitution took effect, the three contending ethnic communities—Serbs, Croats, and Slovenes—struggled for power. Only members of these three groups had political rights. The trio "denied the very existence of Macedonians, Montenegrins, and Bosnian Muslims as distinct ethnic groups in this 'three name [Kingdom].'"[28]

Relations worsened between these three ethnic groups during the 1920s. In 1928 a member of the Serbian National Radical Party (NRS) killed two Croatian deputies. Three other legislators were seriously wounded in the melee. One of them, Stefan Radic, a powerful Croat, later died, leading to unrest and bloodshed against Serbs living in Croatia. The government, for the first time not led by a Serb, resigned.

Consequently, in 1929 King Alexander "concluded that the only way to retain the state was as a personal dictatorship."[29] He annulled the Constitution, dissolved the parliament, and assumed total control of the government. Political parties, freedom of religion, and freedom of speech ended. Reflecting these political and social changes, the monarchy officially became a one-nation state called the Kingdom of Yugoslavia. The King repudiated the existence of ethnic diversity. In the new 1931 Constitution, political associations based on "religious, tribal (ethnic), or regional basis" were once again banned as well as political rights such as freedom of association, assembly, and speech. For the monarch, *Yugoslavism* had to overcome the tribalism of the ethnic communities, especially Serb nationalism.

These actions led to continued unrest and violence in the three regions. In Croatia and Macedonia nationalists were emboldened to organize for actions against the king: in these regions, illegal political action organizations, the Ustashe in Croatia and the Macedonian Revolutionary Organization (VMRO), were formed. A Macedonian terrorist from the VMRO struck hard in 1934, assassinating King Alexander when the monarch visited France. The assassin acted on the orders of the Croat Ustashe leader, Ante Pavelic.[30]

After the assassination, the Croat leaders demanded that Croatia become an autonomous entity and that Yugoslavia switch over to six or seven autonomous ethnic units. Clearly, after 1918, "ethnic differences would not disappear; existing national identities could not be merged into a new Yugoslav identity."[31] The "Croat Question" remained an unresolved issue for Yugoslav politicians until, in August 1939, the King announced a formal decree creating a semi-independent Croatia. According to this "understanding," Croatia annexed one-half of Bosnia but did not provide its Muslims with any rights.[32] It is ironic that the initial success of Yugoslavian nationalists in the twentieth century occurred in Croatia, not Serbia.

In September 1939 World War II began. The Yugoslavian government quickly declared its neutrality. However, by March 1941 Hitler compelled the Yugoslavians to sign the Tripartite Pact, joining that nation to the Axis powers: Germany, Italy, and Japan. Smaller eastern European nations, Bulgaria, Hungary, and Romania, were persuaded to sign the Pact as well.

This action led to demonstrations by anti-Axis Yugoslavs, helped by military men of the British Special Operations Executive, England's spy organization operating in Nazi-occupied nations. That led, in turn, to the Nazi and Italian invasion and the surrender of Yugoslavia's army after eleven days of fighting in April 1941. Yugoslavia, immediately occupied by German, Italian, Hungarian, Bulgarian, and Albanian troops, saw the "independent" state of Croatia formally established by the occupiers. This new puppet state, ruled by Pavelic's Ustashe, consisted of Croatia and Bosnia. Pavelic, with the support of his Italian friend and mentor Mussolini, returned in triumph to his homeland after a decade in exile in Italy.

At the urging of Mussolini, Hitler made Pavelic chieftain of the Croat government. His first speech set the tone for his government. Its primary task, he said, was to "create an *ethnically pure* Croat country across a territory where Croats constituted barely half the population."[33] The major problem for Pavelic was the large Serb minority living in Croatia: 1.9 million out of 6.3 million persons.[34] Pavelic's purification was to be accomplished through the elimination of these alien elements by a process the Ustashe called "cleansing the terrain."[35] (It has, since then, been called by its more common name: *ethnic cleansing*.)

Pavelic's major weapon to cleanse the Serbs from Croatia was his army of terrorist fighters, the Ustashe death squads.

During the war, they "raided Serb villages all over Croatia and Bosnia,"[36] and tortured, deported, and exterminated two million "alien" persons then living there: Jews, Gypsies, the Serbs, and Croats and Muslims who were political opponents of Pavelic.

South of Zagreb, Pavelic established the infamous Jasenovac concentration camp to hold and then murder nearly one million of these "aliens."[37] The killers in the concentration camps used clubs, knives, and other farm implements "because the Ustashe did not want to waste bullets. Their brutality shocked even the Nazis."[38] (In 1992 a Bosnian Serb guard at the Omarska concentration camp told a UN representative that "we don't waste our bullets on them [Bosniaks]. [Here] they have no roof. There is sun and rain, cold nights, and beatings two times a day. We give them no food and water. They will starve like animals. Nightly savage beatings, which maim and kill, reduce [them] from human to nonhuman."[39])

These brutal actions in the Ustashe-controlled Croatia of the 1940s immediately led to the formation of an organized Serbian defense force, the Chetniks (officially known as "the King's Army in the Homeland"), led by Serbian Colonel Dragoljub-Draza Mihailovic. Their primary task throughout the war was to protect ethnic Serbs from extermination by the Croatian Ustashe. The Chetniks saw themselves as Serbian saviors and fought Croats and Muslims to protect their brethren and create the foundation for a Greater Serbia.

To move toward *their* vision of an enlarged and ethnically pure Serbia, the Chetniks also implemented ethnic cleansing of Croats and Muslims living in Serb-controlled regions. "In the name of Greater Serbia, they killed thousands of Muslims and Croats and terrorized the Serbian and Montenegrin people supporting the [Tito-led] partisans."[40]

Both the Ustashe and the Chetniks greatly feared the Yugoslav Partisans, led by Communists. The leaders believed that the Communists were the major threat to their plans to establish an ethnically pure Croatia or a "Greater Serbia."

Finally, spurred on by their concern about the growing power of the Communist Partisans, by the fall of 1941, the Chetnik leadership entered secret talks with the occupying powers, "and this collaboration became open by spring 1942."[41]

The organized resistance by the Communist Party of Yugoslavia, led by Josip Broz, known as Tito,[42] began across Yugoslavia in 1941. Called the National Liberation Movement (NLM), the Communists were the *only* Yugoslav organization that fought against Yugoslavia's occupiers throughout the war, *as well as* battling the Ustashe and the Chetniks (who spent more "time and blood" fighting each other than battling the Axis occupiers).[43] By the spring of 1943, in a major battle between Ustashe, Germany, and Italy and the partisan army, the Communists destroyed Ustashe forces and escaped from the Axis powers.

By the end of the war, even the allies accepted the political and military primacy of the Tito-led Communist partisan forces in Yugoslavia. Tito's slogan, the hallmark of his dictatorial rule, was "Brotherhood and Unity" for Yugoslavians. He successfully dampened—but did not destroy—ethnic nationalism for nearly forty years.[44]

Tito and Communist Party Rule, 1945–1980

By 1945, Tito's partisan armies liberated the entire territory of the former Kingdom of Yugoslavia, including large parts of Croatia and Slovenia ceded to Italy after World War I. The Communist Party took total control of the economy, nationalizing all areas except agriculture, and controlling all intellectual, political, and social life in Yugoslavia. The government nationalized millions of acres; much of the land was taken from ethnic Germans, as well as Catholic and Orthodox Churches and monasteries.

A primary task for the new Communist government called for "silencing certain memories (a strategy of forgetting) and selectively embracing others." To this end, Tito immediately cultivated the new Yugoslav slogan— "brotherhood and unity"—along with a policy of national equality.[45]

Pursuing these goals, Tito initially resorted to mass terror. His military brutally exterminated between 100,000 and 250,000 of their wartime enemies[46]: the Ustashe, the Chetniks, Slovene Home Defenders, and other political opponents of the new Communist regime.[47] In November 1945, he formally established the Yugoslav Federated People's Republic. The new nation consisted of six people's republics: Serbia, Macedonia, Montenegro, Bosnia and Herzegovina, Croatia, and Slovenia. Ironically, the Federation "reinforced national identities" and, after Tito's death in 1980, "the repressed memories surfaced," leading to the ethnic bloodshed of the 1990s.[48]

Unlike the Soviet Union, Tito did not order the collectivization of farming. That same year saw the split between Stalin and Tito that led, in June 1948, to the expulsion of Yugoslavia from the Soviet pact.

By 1953 Yugoslavia ditched the direct administration of the state by the Communist Party and placed management in the hands of local communes in the six federated republics. By the mid-1950s Tito became one of the founders of the movement of nonaligned nations, an association of mostly third world nations that had an impact on international relations throughout the extended Cold War.

During this innovative governing era, a number of the federated republics, especially Serbia, but also Croatia and Slovenia, saw the renewed surge of feelings of autonomy. The memories of World War II, never far from the surface, emerged—as did visions of enlarged, ethnically cleansed nations. Clashes between Croatia, Slovenia, and Serbia became very public: the "Serbs feared that the Catholic North [Croatia and Slovenia] would get too much material support at the expense of the Orthodox South Serbia."[49]

For a decade, 1965–1975, the Communist Party actively purged its ranks, targeting young members of the party for expulsion. The senior leaders, who came to power during and after World War II, believed that the new generation had welcomed too loudly the liberalizing and pro-independence tendencies of the West. Tito started with the young Croatian party members who had begun to talk—again—about the creation of a new independent Croatia. Next, the young Serb party members were targeted because of their very anti-Tito tirades and their talk of a new Serbia. Then the other young party liberals were expelled (but most not murdered) by the central government.

By 1971 Tito reassumed control of all aspects of life in Yugoslavia. Centralism returned as state policy in 1974 in a new constitution. It officially recognized Bosnia's Slavic Muslims as a separate constituent nation.[50] It was clearly an effort to curb the power of resurgent nationalism in Serbia and Croatia. It created a confederation of six equal republics and a collective presidency, with Tito as the new "president for life." In the constitution, the six republics received very limited veto power over the actions of the federal (central) government.

By the end of the 1970s, the Yugoslav economy was bleeding: inflation and mass unemployment took hold (due to the state's inability to produce goods that met the quality standards of the international community, and heightened by a worldwide recession) and drastically changed the lives of Yugoslavians throughout the federation. It was an economic calamity that foreshadowed the economic malaise that went unresolved in Bosnia after 1995.

Furthermore, nationalistic ethnic demands became much louder and bolder during the 1970s. "With the rise of Serbian nationalism in the mid-1980s, [Tito's] system began to break down."[51] Croatian nationalism, too, emerged full-blown in that decade. Mass demonstrations for Croatian independence took place, and violence was present across these two republics.[52] These actions continued unabated after Marshall Tito's death in 1980.

Tito's Death and the Dissolution of Yugoslavia, 1980–1990

Tito's death on May 4, 1980, "spelled the beginning of the end for Yugoslavia." There was no one in the republic who could successfully lead the country. "The state now had no leader who could, with charisma, paper over regional differences in the state and in interethnic relations."[53] Throughout the 1980s, the revolving presidency was unable to dampen down the frictions that blossomed in the post-Tito era. After Tito's death, the "importance of ethnicity [would over the decade] swell to grotesque proportions."[54]

Further moving Yugoslavia toward dissolution was the continuing economic travail in the nation. "More than a decade of austerity and declining living standards corroded the social fabric and the rights and securities that individuals and families had come to rely on. Normal political conflicts became constitutional conflicts and then a crisis of the state itself among politicians who were unwilling to compromise."[55]

As early as 1981, there were local rebellions within Kosovo's (majority) ethnic Albanian population. Internal dissension and intrigue continued throughout the decade. In response to the Kosovo demands for autonomy and the resurfacing of Croat nationalism, Serb nationalists stridently wrangled with their opponents during the chaotic decade. Further increasing the move toward dissolution, legislation passed during 1989 by the federal government allowed Slovenia the right to secede from the federation.

In 1986 a secret memorandum prepared by the Serbian

34

Academy of Arts and Sciences triggered sensational and adverse reactions from the Yugoslav Federation members, including some Serbian leaders. Unnervingly, it had its roots in the 1844 secret memorandum that laid the blueprint for a greater Serbian nation. The 1986 document expressed a "deep concern" and condemnation of the existing Yugoslav political, economic, and legal systems. There is no collective nation anymore; instead, there are eight territories and seven of them continually discriminate against the Serb republic and the hundreds of thousands of ethnic Serbs living in Kosovo, Croatia, and Bosnia.

"Separatism and nationalism are active on the social scene," the memo stated, leading to the spread "of apathy and bitterness" among the public. This reality has "driven the ethnic nations further from one another to a critical degree." Serbia is the target of the less economically developed republics in the Yugoslav Federation. The memo warned its readers that unless there was an end to the "physical, political, legal, and cultural genocide perpetrated against the Serbian population," Yugoslavia would disintegrate into civil war, out of which a renewed and (once again) a Greater Serbia would emerge.

This memo was a watershed document in the disintegration of Tito's Yugoslavia. The memory of a gloried past returned with clarity and stridency. The document concluded with the authors calling for increased Serbian nationalism and the reemergence of a "Greater Serbia":

> Complete national and cultural integrity of the Serbian people is their historic and democratic right, *no matter in which republic or province they may find themselves living.* . . . In order to have a future in the international family of cultured and civilized nations, the Serbian *nation must have an opportunity to find itself again and become a historical agent, must re-acquire an awareness of its historical and spiritual being, must look its*

economic and cultural interests square in the eyes, and must find a modern social and national program that will inspire this generation and generations to come.[56] (my emphasis)

While local Communist parties in the federation trashed the memo as incendiary rantings, it was a monumental harbinger of events that would occur in less than five years. Bosniaks saw the 1986 memo as a mortal threat to their life. For them, the document was "as histrionic as it [was] racist and inaccurate."[57]

The Serbian leader who emerged during this time was Slobodan Milosevic.[58] Elected president of Serbia in 1987, by 1988 Milosevic began to quash the autonomy movement in the Serbian province of Kosovo as well as develop a strategy for assuming total control of Yugoslavia.

Milosevic, while publicly disavowing the 1986 memo, grasped the significance of its message to the Serb nation and ethnic Serbs living across Yugoslavia. In 1987 he began to initiate concrete political actions to "re-acquire an awareness of [Serbia's] historical and spiritual being."[59]

For many scholars, the second critical turning point in the disintegration of Yugoslavia came in June 1989. Milosevic's plan to gather total power for Serbia in a disintegrating Yugoslavia was to radicalize and unify the Serbs across Yugoslavia into a single political unit "which would either dominate Yugoslavia or break it apart."[60]

Milosevic's strategy—mobilization of the ethnic Serbs living outside Serbia—in order for him to seize control unfolded with a June 28, 1989, speech he gave at Gazimestan in Kosovo to the more than one million Serbs in attendance and listening on radio and television. The event marked the six hundredth anniversary of the Serb *defeat* by the Turks.

A defiant Milosevic began his speech[61] with electrifying words that trumpeted the rebirth of the idea of a great

Serbia. He told his countrymen that they were "the chosen people," a "celestial people." His speech was televised across Yugoslavia and "nationalist euphoria" swept over [Yugoslavia] in response to Milosevic's words.[62]

He then began using three tactics to try to gain total power in a Greater Serbia. Employing them beginning in 1990, he assured the destruction of Yugoslavia.

1. Use the media[63]—television, radio, and the press—to *radicalize* the Serb minorities in Croatia and Bosnia by using provocative language and misinformation to profanely label the Croats ("Ustashe Terror") and the Bosniaks ("Islamic Fundamentalists" and "Turks"). Such tactics struck fear into the ethnic Serbs living in those two republics. They also led to the radicalization of the Croats and the Muslims. Very quickly, these two ethnic populations saw the Serbs as dangerous, and they became eager to eliminate their newly avowed enemy. This reemergent hatred is clearly present in the comments of a Croatian civilian to his neighbor, an ethnic Serb, in 1991: "You never expected us to be the ones to kill you. We are happy to surprise you."[64]

2. Instigate gun battles and skirmishes between ethnic Serbs and Croat soldiers in Serb-majority villages that, hopefully, would lead to a Croatian crackdown in those villages, which would further radicalize the ethnic Serbs living in Croatia.

3. With that as a foundation, foment wider military clashes between the Yugoslav military (primarily populated by Serb soldiers and officers) and the Croat military, in which the Croats would be defeated and Serbia would gain control of Croatia.[65]

Milosevic also employed this three-pronged strategy to mobilize the ethnic Serbs living in Bosnia by labeling the

Bosniaks as Islamic Fundamentalist terrorists. Even though this message was absolutely false,[66] it heightened the fears of the ethnic Serbs living in Bosnia.

Milosevic's erstwhile friend (but afterward his adversary) was the leader of the other nationalistic movement in the dissolving state of Yugoslavia, the Croatian ultranationalist, Franjo Tudjman, the president of Croatia in 1991.[67]

Both leaders were powerful speakers and loudly encouraged their ethnic followers in Serbia, Croatia, Kosovo, and Bosnia to join the movement for a "Greater Croatia" or a "Greater Serbia" at the expense of the other indigenous ethnic groups in Yugoslavia, chiefly the Bosniaks.

In response, the Bosniaks, who made up over 40 percent of the population in Bosnia, formed a nationalistic party of their own, the Party for Democratic Action, led by Alija Izetbegovic.[68] Mr. Izetbegovic built a Muslim political organization in 1990, as the old Yugoslavia continued on its path to dissolution and into the maelstrom of competing nationalisms. After winning elections late that year, President Izetbegovic led his republic toward independence.

His actions were immediately supported by Western nations but not by the ethnic Serbs, who made up some one-third of the pre-1992-war population of Bosnia.[69] His greatest fear was the "tearing apart of Bosnia by Croatia and Serbia in their efforts to create more expansive [empires]."[70]

Immediately after Izetbegovic's action, the Bosnian Serb nationalists countered by creating a party of their own, the Serbian Democratic Party, led by Radovan Karadzic. Like Milosevic, Karadzic was a true believer and advocate for a "Greater Serbia." He believed that "the need to avenge Serb deaths during WWII would justify anything his people might do. In his mind, the blood on the Serbs' hands during the war had been justified by the Ustashe genocide. He said, 'The Serbs are endangered again [but] the Serbs are ready for war. If someone forces them to live as a national minority, they are ready for war. *The memory of those events [during WWII] is still a living memory, a terrible living memory.* The terror has survived fifty years. The feeling is present still because they won't allow us to bury the dead.'" (my emphasis)[71]

The horrific events that occurred in World War II became rallying points for the fighting forces in the 1990s. Additionally, for the Serb nationalists, the memory of the agony of defeat by the Turks in 1389 Kosovo reemerged. In 1991, the first of the Balkan wars, between Croatia and Serbia, began.[72]

The Balkan Wars Begin, I: Croatia versus Serbia, 1991–1995

Tudjman became president of Croatia in an election in which he praised the actions of the Croatian Ustashe during World War II. The words inflamed Milosevic and Serbs across Yugoslavia. Tudjman immediately placed his nationalistic ideas into the new constitution. The new Croatian coat of arms bore a striking resemblance to the World War II fascist Ustashe symbol.

All references to Serbia and Serbs in the old constitution were deleted in the 1990 document. Serbs were "systematically removed from all professional and bureaucratic positions. Thousands lost their jobs. Croatian Serbs were frightened by steps taken to secede from Yugoslavia. Old Ustashe fighters [returned] to the state "and the Serbs in Croatia started a similar process of self-organization and preparation for self-defense [with the active assistance of Milosevic]."[73]

In early 1991, Milosevic's strategy led to ethnic, religious, and racial tensions between the Croat police and ethnic Serbs living in Croatia. They quickly "escalated into violence as the country slowly drifted into civil war."[74] It became impossible to fix these interethnic problems through peaceful negotiations.

By late June 1991, both Slovenia and Croatia declared their independence. Serbia's immediate response was implementation of Milosevic's final segment of his strategy: Yugoslavia/Serbian Army (JNA) military actions to protect the ethnic Serbians living in Croatia. War broke out the following month. Only 12 percent of Croatia's population were ethnic Serbs. Only in the Krajina enclave in northern Croatia did Serbs form a majority. However, given Milosevic's push to create a "Greater Serbia," Croat-Serb irregulars, backed by arms and Yugoslavian troops from Serbia itself, seized control of about 30 percent of Croatia's territory. "Ethnic cleansing," the World War II phrase, was reintroduced by journalists in 1991 to describe the Serb policy that drove out or massacred Croatian villagers from this area of Croatia.[75]

The policy of terrorism began after the shelling ceased. Serbs executed hundreds of Croats, civilian and military, wounded, and those who surrendered. "Serb irregulars pulled men in civilian clothes out of groups of shell-shocked refugees and shot them dead on the spot."[76] After their successful siege of Vukovar (the city surrendered to the JNA and Croat-Serbs in November 1991), "Serb forces marched into the city hospital, brought out several hundred wounded men and women [soldiers and hospital staff], and executed them, burying them in one of the war's first mass graves."[77] They did this while nearby, the ICRC representative argued with a JNA officer in an unsuccessful effort to gain access to the hospital![78]

Clea Koff, a twenty-something forensic anthropologist, was part of the initial forensic team that unearthed the mortal remains of both patients and hospital staff murdered by the Bosnian Serb forces. The UN Commission of Experts, in 1992, asked the Physicians for Human Rights (PHR), an NGO, to form a team to examine the rubbish pit where the bodies were buried; however, "the forensic team was run off the site at gunpoint by local Serbian authorities.

The only solution was for the UN to protect the grave from tampering until a forensic team could return in safety. Soldiers ended up guarding the site for four years, until exhumation began in 1996."[79]

Once work began at the site (Ovcara), Koff and the team found multiple layers of bodies. They discovered medical staff, whose mortal remains were still clothed in green medical smocks. "Also, patients with casts and patients with catheters still attached were found by the forensics staff. Others were found with medical gauze wrapped around skulls; some were wearing pajamas, one had x-ray films tucked in his bathrobe. Thinking about that man makes me cry," Koff wrote in her book, "but at the time it was as if he had left us a note."[80]

By 1993 a fragile cease-fire was brokered between the two nations. However, after reequipping their army—with the help of German and American political and military leaders—in the summer of 1995, Croatian forces crossed the cease-fire line and recaptured the Krajina region. The troops drove out some 170,000 ethnic Serbs, who fled to Bosnia and Serbia. Hundreds of others were found with bullet holes in their heads or in mass unmarked graves, leading some foreign observers to question whether Croatia also was practicing "ethnic cleansing." Not everyone believed President Tudjman when he said he was doing all he could to stop the killings and punish those responsible.[81]

The Second Balkan War: Bosnia versus Serbia, 1992–1995

The Balkan wars of the 1990s were the "product of bad, even criminal, political leaders [especially Serbia's Milosevic] who encouraged ethnic confrontation for personal, political, and financial gain. They led their people into a war."[82] For Milosevic, Karadzic, Mladic, and others who dreamed of a Greater Serbia, that meant that Muslims must be eradicated from all Serb territories. According to one of the devotees of this Serbian *lebensraum*, Vladimir Srebov, the solution was stark: More than 50 percent had to be murdered, a small number converted to orthodoxy, and an even smaller number of Muslims—those with money—would be allowed to buy their lives and emigrate to safety in Turkey.[83] According to General Mladic's military deputy, General Manojlo Milovanovic (testifying at Mladic's ICTY trial in The Hague in September 2013), the Bosnian Serb military leader told the Bosnian Serb political leaders the day before the war against the Bosniaks began in May 1992: "We cannot ethnically cleanse, we don't have a sieve to sift so that only Serbs can stay, and others leave. . . . I don't know how you, Mr. Karadzic and Mr. Krajisnik (the Bosnian Serb political leaders), will explain this to the world. This is genocide, people."[84]

By 2007, after reviewing 240,000 pieces of information, an international team of experts concluded that more than 100,000 Bosnian citizens were killed during the 1992–1995 war: 83 percent of the dead were Bosniaks, 10 percent Bosnian Serbs, and 5 percent Bosnian Croats.[85]

The war became inevitable after February 29–March 1, 1992, when a referendum resulted in 63 percent of the population voting for independence from Yugoslavia, and the establishment of a multiethnic Republic of Bosnia-Herzegovina. Nearly all the ethnic Serbs living in Bosnia boycotted the election.

On the floor of the parliament, after the vote, the bitter leader of the Bosnian Serbs, Radovan Karadzic, angrily threatened the Muslims with war and the destruction of their way of life: "I warn you, you'll drag Bosnia down to Hell. You Muslims aren't ready for war—you'll face extinction."[86] (Radovan Karadzic and General Ratko Mladic became the leaders of the Bosnian Serbs. Mladic, a general in the JNA, was picked by Slobodan Milosevic in May 1992 to take command of the Bosnian Serb army and paramilitaries.[87])

The new president of Bosnia, Alija Izetbegovic, followed Karadzic to the rostrum. He said, "His words and his manners show why others refuse to remain in this Yugoslavia. The kind of Yugoslavia that Mr. Karadzic wants, nobody else wants anymore, nobody except perhaps the Serbs. This Yugoslavia and the manners of Karadzic are simply hated by the peoples of Yugoslavia, by Slovenes, Croats, Macedonians, Albanians, Hungarians, Muslims. . . . I solemnly state that the Muslims will defend themselves with great determination and that they will survive."[88]

The new republic, recognized by the European Union and the United States in early April 1992, joined the United Nations in May 1992. It had a short life; it ended in November 1995 with the signing of the Dayton Accords.

On May 12, 1992, the Bosnian war began when the Yugoslav Army (JNA), consisting mostly of Serb and Macedonian troops, began shelling Muslim cities in the new republic. These JNA forces were joined in these military actions by Karadzic's brutal Bosnian Serb paramilitaries.[89] They were commanded by General Mladic.

Immediately, the ethnic Serbs in Bosnia, with the support of the Yugoslav Army and the president of Serbia, Slobodan Milosevic, announced the creation of their own republic, the Bosnian-Serb Republika Srpska (RS), and their own army, the Army of the Serb Republic (VRS).

In May 1992 the combined Serb armies began their attacks on Muslim villages in eastern Bosnia. There also began the forty-three-month siege of Sarajevo (May 1992–November 1995). Nearly sixty thousand Bosnian Serbs fled Sarajevo as soon as the bombardment began.[90] The siege took on the character of other brutal sieges throughout history. One seventeen-year-old student told a reporter for the BBC: "I ate grass for four years. I still can't eat meat or butter or anything which is hard to digest 15 years later."[91]

General Mladic told his gunners in the hills above

Sarajevo at the beginning of the bombardment: "Shoot at slow intervals until I order you to stop. Target Muslim neighborhoods—not many Serbs live there. Shell them until they're on the edge of madness."[92]

Death squads terrorized the Muslim civilians in these areas, "executing them in a bloodbath, going house to house, robbing and killing all Muslims they found. Bodies were dumped in the Drina River."[93]

Another strategic terror policy introduced in the war was the sexual abuse and rape of tens of thousands of Bosniak women by Bosnian Serb military. Until this war, sexual abuse and rape as a violation of the Geneva and genocide treaties "had been ignored in all international instruments," said Gabrielle Kirk McDonald, former ICTY president. The Hague Tribunal "played a historical role in the criminal prosecution of sexual abuse committed during the wars in the former Yugoslavia and paved the way for other courts throughout the world to process such crimes. I believe that what the ICTY has done, firstly, by including rape among crimes against humanity, and, secondly, by criminally prosecuting the perpetrators and developing practices against sexual abuse, has led to a situation whereby the leaders in those conflicts were warned that the rules had changed. This is significant progress."[94]

Rapes, sexual abuse, and other crimes against civilians are crimes against humanity, or genocide if it is proven that these crimes were intentionally committed by the military to eliminate, in whole or in part, a targeted population based on their ethnicity or religion. The task of the prosecutor of the international criminal tribunal, in this situation, the ICTY, is to indict and convict those charged with the crimes that fall under the ICTY's jurisdiction: war crimes, crimes against humanity, and genocide. For conviction of a war crime, the prosecutor, using evidence collected by forensic experts, has to provide data that establishes that the killings by combatants were unlawful because they exceeded the scope of immunity provided to lawful belligerents under the treaties and conventions enumerating both lawful and unlawful acts of combatants. To convict a defendant charged with crimes against humanity or genocide, the prosecutor must establish that *civilians* were the target of the attack (either before or during otherwise lawful combat), that the attack was intentional, widespread, or systematic, and that it was aimed at destroying, "in whole or in part," a religious or ethnic minority group.

During the Bosnian war, rapes and other sexual abuses occurred daily. Young women were raped, as well as their mothers and grandmothers. A Bosniak woman from Foca gave chilling testimony before The Hague about the rape that had occurred when she had been fifteen years old: "After having finished it, I mean rape, he sat down and lit a cigarette. He said he might be able to do more, much more, but he would not do it for the time being, because I was of the same age as his daughter."[95]

Since the ICTY began its trial work, the Prosecutor's Office "has charged 78, out of a total of 161 indictees, with sexual crimes."[96] In another criminal trial before the ICTY, E.M., a witness for the prosecution, testifying against Veselin "Batko" Vlahovic, said that Vlahovic committed "psychological abuse [against E.M.'s] father-in-law and his sister-in-law, who was seven months pregnant at the time, and the indictee threatened he would cut their throats, then he plundered their apartment, and then he raped the pregnant sister-in-law in anther room."[97]

By the end of May 1992, the VRS controlled nearly 70 percent of Bosnia. In 1993 Bosnian Muslim forces found themselves in control only in central Bosnia—in a small triangle touching Sarajevo, Tuzla, and Tranik. By 1993 Bosnian Croats occupied the western portion of the country.

The war settled into a stalemate except that the *ethnic*

cleansing of Bosnian Muslims continued until the war ended in 1995. In town after town, the Serbs methodically drove Muslims out, executing many of the men and boys and forcing the remainder to flee to another Muslim village in those areas of Bosnia still retained by the Muslims. Once the Muslim residents fled, ethnic Serbs moved into the now-empty homes and apartments.

In the three years of war, over half of the nation's 4.3 million people were driven from their homes; over one million were internally displaced while the rest became refugees in other European nations. In no city or town in Bosnia did the prewar ethnic composition remain the same. All mosques and Catholic churches in the areas occupied by Bosnian Serbs were destroyed, many replaced by Orthodox churches.[98]

In 1995, before Srebrenica's tragic fall, a classified CIA report concluded that the Bosnian Serbs carried out 90 percent of all war crimes and crimes against humanity in the 1991–1995 Balkan wars. They were the only warring party to attempt "systematically to eliminate all traces of other ethnic groups from their territory."[99]

The UN brokered an agreement between the warring forces on April 21, 1993, announcing that the demilitarization by both sides "had been a success." However, the Serbs never demilitarized. Instead, the Serb armies around Srebrenica in eastern Bosnia "constantly attacked neighboring Bosnian Muslim villages." They destroyed more than four hundred villages around Srebrenica in 1992 alone with at least eleven thousand Muslims killed in the Drina River valley.[100]

From 1993 to 1995 Serb military forces from heavily fortified villages surrounding Srebrenica forced forty thousand Bosnian Muslims to move into Srebrenica ghetto areas with little or no means of survival. This siege of Srebrenica— sniper shootings, bombings, air attacks, cutting off the water supply, not allowing medical and food supplies into the besieged city—continued until spring 1995. A doctor working for the World Health Organization (who), Simon Mardel, in Srebrenica during the siege, wrote, "People are completely trapped. The water from higher up in the valley is now cut off. The present situation can only be described as an impending holocaust."[101]

By 1994, however, new events changed the character of the Bosnian war. While the Bosnian Serbs still had about eighty thousand troops and controlled 70 percent of Bosnia, the Bosniaks now had three times that many men under arms. In addition, the Bosniaks were now getting military hardware from America through transshipments to Zagreb, Croatia, via a secret airlift. By the end of 1994, tons of equipment from Turkey, Saudi Arabia, and Iran had reached the Bosniak military. Both the Croat and Bosnian armies began to plan offensive operations to regain territory seized by the Serbs.[102]

The Bosnian Serb response, in July 1995, was the next, final phase in their three-year siege of Srebrenica and other small towns populated by Muslims located in misnamed "safe havens" created by the un in 1993. The new plan was a frontal attack on these aberrant Muslim entities in the midst of heavily Bosnian Serb population sites in eastern Bosnia.

"Ethnic Cleansing": The Tragedy of Srebrenica, July 1995

In 1995 there was an "anomaly" deep in the heart of Serb-occupied eastern Bosnia: the presence of Bosnian Muslim enclaves, so-called un-labeled "safe havens" established in 1993. On July 10, 1995, General Mladic took care of the glitch. He ordered his troops to attack the three Muslim enclaves—Srebrenica, Zepa, and Gorazde—surrounded by Serb forces but labeled "safe havens" with un military personnel located there. He told them: "It is going to be a *meza* (a long, luscious feast). There will be blood up to your knees."[103]

The Muslim residents relied on the promises of the UN that the peacekeepers would protect them from harm. That did not happen. The soldiers were outnumbered and outgunned by the Bosnian Serb military. Requests by the Dutch commander for NATO airstrikes to halt the Serb offensive were rejected. "The victims had put their trust in international protection. But we, the international community, let them down. This was a colossal, collective failure," said Javier Solana, the European Union's chief of foreign policy.[104]

The UN peacekeepers, UNPROFOR soldiers from Denmark, stood by impotently while the killings took place. A Bosniak civic woman's NGO contended that the UN soldiers "in fact assisted the [Serbs] separate unarmed men and boys from their families and bus them to execution sites."[105]

Two days after the Bosnian Serb forces and paramilitary groups, under Mladic's leadership, began the massacre, the "outnumbered and poorly equipped Dutch UN peacekeepers—or *Dutchbat*—bowed to General Mladic's demands and forced many Muslim families who had sought refuge on their base out of the compound."[106] (In 2011 a Dutch appeals court overturned a 2008 lower court ruling that the government bore no responsibility for the 1995 genocide. The appellate court judges said that Dutch military and political leaders were in "effective control" of their troops in Srebrenica. Therefore, the judges concluded, "the State is responsible for the death of these men as *Dutchbat* should not have turned these men over to the Serbs."[107])

In July 2014, in what has been called a "bittersweet judgment," another Dutch court ruled that the Netherlands *was liable only* for the killings of more than three hundred Bosniak men and boys who were *forcibly ousted* from the Dutchbat compound by its military and killed by the Serbs, and that *only* the surviving family members of the three hundred expelled Bosniaks were entitled to compensation from the country.[108]

According to Ambassador Holbrooke, General Mladic "decided to eliminate the enclaves from the map in order to secure the entire eastern portion of Bosnia for the Serbs. . . . The biggest single mass murder in Europe since WWII took place, while the outside world did nothing to stop the tragedy."[109]

Nearly nine thousand Muslim men and boys were exterminated in a little more than seven days by the Serb military in July 1995.[110] General Radislav Krstic, the deputy commander of the Drina Corps of the ARS, told his troops in a radio broadcast: "You must kill everyone. We don't need anyone alive."[111] Another Serb officer counseled his men to "kill them slowly. We don't need any surprises. Surround them [on the road] and kill them slowly."[112]

Another thirty thousand Bosnian Muslims, mostly women and children, were expelled and sent to Tuzla in the Bosnian Muslim area. The Bosnian Serb soldiers raped many thousands of Muslim women. Srebrenica's missing are almost 40 percent of the total number of civilians who disappeared during the war.[113] Many women died during and after enduring multiple rapes, while some committed suicide or went mad.[114] The pages of the ICTY's ruling in *Prosecutor v Krstic*, August 2001, substantiate the dreadfulness: "Bosnian Muslim refugees could see the rapes, but could do nothing because of Serb soldiers standing nearby. Other people heard women screaming, or saw women being dragged away. Several individuals were so terrified that they committed suicide by hanging themselves."[115]

The ICTY found beyond a reasonable doubt that the vast majority of those killed were not killed in combat; Bosnian Serbs cold-bloodedly executed them. The acts were the outcome of a well-planned and coordinated operation ordered by General Mladic. One witness told a Human Rights Watch (HRW) reporter the following horror scene he witnessed in Srebrenica: "The Serbs picked out Muslims, interrogated them and made them dig pits. . . . They would just line them up and shoot them into the pits. . . . At dawn, a bulldozer arrived and dug up a pit and buried about 400 men alive. The men were encircled by Chetniks; whoever tried to escape was shot."[116]

The ICTY judges concluded that the killing of thousands of Muslim civilians constituted genocide. The extermination of men and boys and the rape of hundreds of Muslim women in the Srebrenica area was the first legally established case of genocide in Europe, acknowledged by both the ICTY and the International Court of Justice (ICJ). In sentencing General Krstic to forty-six years for his genocidal actions in Srebrenica, the presiding judge Almiro Rodrigues concluded: "In July 1995, Gereral Krstic, you committed evil." The Appeals Chamber of the ICTY, three years later in 2004, reaffirmed the tribunal's conclusions while reducing the penalty to thirty-five years.[117] Presiding Judge Theodor Meron said, "By seeking to eliminate a part of the Bosnian Muslims, the Bosnian Serb forces committed genocide. They targeted for extinction the forty thousand Bosnian Muslims living in Srebrenica, a group which was emblematic of the Bosnian Muslims in general."[118]

The prosecutors' allocution of the genocidal behavior of the Bosnian Serb leaders and their soldiers presented hard evidence. One example presented was a transcript of a telephone conversation between Bosnian Serb general Krstic and Colonel Beara on July 15, 1995. Beara asked for more troops to execute the Muslim men. "I don't know what to do. I mean it. There are still 3,500 'parcels' that I have to 'distribute' and I have no solution." Krstic's reply, "Fuck it, I'll see what I can do." Extra soldiers arrived immediately for the killing work. From a document produced at the trial:

BALKAN NATIONALISM

"The very next day, men from the Bratunac Brigade arrived to assist members of the 10th Sabotage Detachment with the executions at the Branjevo Military Farm." These mass killings took place there and at least at eight other sites in the Srebrenica area.[119]

As of July 2013, at least eight members of the Tenth Sabotage Battalion had admitted guilt in the ICTY to their genocidal actions and had been sentenced to prison terms, although not as harsh as Krstic's sentence. The first to admit guilt, Drazen Erdemovic, told the court, "I had to do it. If I refused it, they would have killed me with those people. . . . They would have told me: 'If you are feeling sorry, stand with them so we can kill you, too.'"[120]

One of Erdemovic's codefendants, Franc Kos, described the event in his testimony before the ICTY. It was a chilling account of the genocide: "We were killing the men in groups of ten who the military police took off the buses. Prisoners from the first two buses had their hands tied, and I think the others had their eyes bandaged. It took us one hour to shoot the people from one bus."[121] (As of July 2013, five of the eight men, including Erdemovic and Kos, were serving a total of 112 years of imprisonment for their murder of Bosniak civilians in Srebrenica.[122])

An appalling footnote to the Srebrenica horror: A CIA official stated that the executions at Srebrenica were seen live on television screens at the CIA's Langley, Virginia, headquarters.[123]

Most of the dead were *not* battlefield casualties. When the bodies were finally found and exhumed, many hundreds of human remains had blindfolds, or had their hands tied behind their backs. Furthermore, the ICTY judges found that some of the dead were handicapped elderly men and young children. As Momir Nikolic, the Bosnian Serb Deputy Commander for Security and Intelligence, told the Court, the Geneva Conventions did not exist in Bosnia in the 1990s.

"Do you really think that in an operation where [thousands] of people were set aside, captured, and killed that somebody was adhering to the Geneva Conventions? First of all, they were captured, killed, and then buried, exhumed once again, buried again. . . . Nobody adhered to the Geneva Conventions or the rules and regulations."[124]

The slaughter of thousands of Bosniaks in July 1995 became worldwide news. Earlier exposés of the existence of Serb concentration camps triggered a global outcry and led to outside involvement by the ICRC and Physicians for Human Rights to mitigate the suffering and dying of the inmates.

The Srebrenica mini-holocaust moved the West, especially U.S. president Bill Clinton, to force the warring parties—Serbs, Muslims, Bosnian Serbs, and Croats—to meet at the airbase in Dayton, Ohio, work out a peace settlement and, finally, accept the Dayton Peace Accords of November 1995.[125] The final document created the nation of Bosnia and Herzegovina with two entities: the Federation of Bosnia and Herzegovina, consisting primarily of Bosnian Croats (41 percent) and Bosniaks (53 percent); and the Bosnian Serb entity, Republika Srpska.

The next phase after the peace deal concluded, following weeks of stressful bargaining and pressure,[126] is one still going on two decades after Dayton: the grim task of locating the more than thirty thousand persons, mostly civilian, mostly Bosnian Muslim civilians, buried throughout the war-torn nation.

The Graves of the Missing

According to a 2010 UN report, since 1995 there have been no less than five thousand locations of mass graves found by the various commissions for missing persons (in Serbia, Croatia, the Federation, and Republika Srpska). Each year the "largest mass grave" is discovered and announced in the press.[127]

Some of them have been located in lakes fed by the rivers in Bosnia, especially the Drina River. In August 2010 more than sixty partial skeletons were found in Lake Perucac, evidently killed in 1992 near Visegrad (one thousand Bosniaks disappeared when Serb forces occupied the town). Some of the bodies, thrown into the Drina, drifted into the lake where they lay undiscovered until workers drained the lake eighteen years later.[128] Other human remains were dumped into caves, quarries, and mountain crevices, some of them eighty meters deep. Many mass graves were hurriedly established, and then bodies removed and reburied—often more than two times in order to hide evidence of war crimes and genocide.

Nearly twenty-five thousand human remains were discovered at these locations. Most of these sites were in the once-heavily Muslim-populated eastern Bosnia, around Foca, Cerska, Visegrad, Vlasenica, Rudo, Cajnice, Zvornik, Srebrenica, and Bratunac. However, concluded the report, "finding mass graves is getting harder as time goes by."[129] There are gravesites still undiscovered two decades after the executions and disappearances occurred. Unfortunately, as Amor Masovic told me, as the years go by, there are fewer pieces of information about the location of the graves and the missing people.

Finding the mortal remains of the missing is the necessary first phase in the herculean work efforts by forensic professionals. After that happens, it is up to these forensic scientists to identify the missing and determine the cause of death. These are time-consuming and difficult tasks.

Chapter 3 examines both the problems and the methods employed by the searchers in the field and in the morgue to resolve them. It will also examine the major organizations, governmental and nongovernmental, involved in the process of finding and identifying the missing—and turning over to the ICTY and state criminal prosecutors evidence of war crimes and crimes against humanity committed by those who murdered civilians and prisoners of war.

THREE

Finding, Exhuming, and Identifying the Human Remains in Bosnia

The families of the missing are today living remains of stolen lives.

—EMIR SULJAGIC, 2000

All [forensic] investigations are directed towards [two] ends: *judicial investigation* (for possible war crimes or genocide) and *humanitarian relief.*

—MARGARET COX, AMBIKA FLAVEL, IAN HANSON, JOANNA LAVER, AND ROLAND WESSLING, 2008

We come now to the essential tasks that drive the men and women who have come from two dozen nations to do forensic work in Bosnia: finding the missing, exhuming the remains, and identifying them. As noted earlier, these and other notoriously difficult and frustrating tasks[1] must be dealt with satisfactorily if the 1995 creation by the Dayton peace delegates, the state of Bosnia and Herzegovina, is to survive.

True reconciliation in this region will not be realized until the missing are found, identified, and properly buried by their surviving family members. Further, there can be no real and lasting peace until those who have committed crimes against humanity, war crimes, or genocide are brought to justice at The Hague and in Bosnia's state courts. Two decades after the signing of the Dayton Peace Accord, hatred, suspicion, massive government corruption, and obstructionism exist in Bosnia and Herzegovina.

Although there was, in 1992, an initial effort by UN authorities, it was not until after the fighting ended in 1995 that forensic professionals began work in the field and in mortuaries examining the mortal remains and reporting the findings to prosecutors and humanitarian organizations. It is extremely dangerous work that these searchers engage in for prosecutors and surviving family members desperate for information about the disappeared.

Every phase of forensic work in war zones "incurs a number of potential risks—injury, health, psychological, and security hazards—to the safety of team members."[2] Risk assessment of the three forensic work phases—finding a site, site excavation and evidence recovery, and mortuary operations—*must* continue until the site and the mortuary facility are closed. Every forensics team that operates in the field has a health and safety officer whose primary task is responsibility for ensuring the health, safety, and security of the team; team leaders continuously point out to their colleagues that "every member must take personal responsibility for his/her own safety."[3]

The First Phase: Where Are They?

There are few frustrations for the forensics personnel worse than not knowing where the graves are located. In 2015 [less than] ten thousand disappeared souls are "still resting in unknown graves in the Bosnian forests and mountains."[4] Generally, there are both noninvasive ways (for example, witnesses and cadaver dogs) and invasive ways (trenching for a possible site, test plots, area stripping) to locate the graves. Forensic teams use both tactics although their wish is to hear about a grave site from a human source.

Finding the missing, however, is extremely difficult, for there are a number of basic obstructions placed in front of the searchers: lack of information about the locations of the gravesites (which are known only by the perpetrators of the crimes); political obstruction; burial and reburial of mortal remains of victims; and the dangers facing searchers working in the field.

DEARTH OF INFORMANTS. The prime source of information about the location of the gravesite is the anonymous person—military or civilian—who knows where a mass grave is and informs officials of its whereabouts. However, many persons who know of the grave locations withhold that information from the families and from the searchers. For those who do inform, the act is dangerous. Amor Masovic told me about one informant who had to leave his home, in Foca, an RS village, travel to Sarajevo, and mail the letter to the authorities. The person simply could not risk sending the letter from his local post office to the searchers because of fear of retribution from his ethnic Serb neighbors.

This source of information, not always accurate because of "emotional stress, [or] seasonal changes in topography or landmarks that may have been destroyed," is "still the most important and reliable source of information for general or specific site location of the grave."[5]

These few revealers, ethnic Serbs or Croats who fought and killed Bosniaks, are probably motivated to act, as Masovic said, because their "conscience prevails, [they] are willing to disclose information about a mass grave, and thus help is given. They do it [basically] to help themselves and release a terrible burden and a terrible secret."[6]

Other information about missing gravesites comes from witnesses who stumble across a possible gravesite location, and those who reveal critical information about site location when testifying at criminal trials at The Hague (ICTY) or in Bosnia's criminal courts. On occasion, the ICTY's prosecutor negotiates plea bargains with defendants in exchange for the locations of gravesites.[7] (This plea bargaining has angered Bosniaks because of the leniency offered to the killers for the vital information.)

Furthermore, the searchers have received less and less information from human sources in recent years about potential gravesites. Seldom does this critically important information reach government investigators. Because of its rarity, when confirmed, the information immediately becomes national news.

For example, a very recent (2013) "discovery" of a mass gravesite containing the remains of Bosniak and ethnic Croat victims in the Tomasica mine near Prijedor appeared in newscasts across Bosnia. Headlines blasted out the news: "An Insider Reveals a Mass Grave near Prijedor." According to press reports, a former Bosnian Serb Army soldier provided the information. The story categorized the find as a "primary" burial site, one of the "biggest graves" ever found in the region, containing *dozens* of mortal remains buried seven meters deep in the ground. "It was hidden under artificial layers of soil. Following detailed digging, a layer a few meters thick and consisting of piled human remains, was discovered."[8] The spokesperson provided no details about the informant. This is simply a standard operating protocol of the office of the prosecutor.

As the fieldwork at this site continued in 2014, forensic archeologists came across the remains of *hundreds* more Bosniaks and Croats in newly uncovered deep mine shafts. It was a tremendous discovery. An MPI spokesperson excitedly proclaimed that there were "435 [new] victims, 275 were complete bodies."[9] The fieldwork continues at the site; the newly found mortal remains added to the hundreds of bodies awaiting autopsy in the mortuary's cavernous refrigerated holding room.

However, two decades after the murders, burials, and reburials, site location information from informants remains exceedingly rare; that reality troubles forensic professionals and prosecutors and devastates the survivors. As a Bosnian Muslim widow said, "There are many people today who know the location of gravesites and say nothing. They cannot conceive of the extent of pain caused by their silence."[10]

A basic reason for their silence is that "they do not sympathize enough with the families of the victims to make an anonymous call and tell us where we could find the remains." Sanja Mulac, a researcher for the Bosnia Missing Persons Institute (M P I), then said she "personally had close contact with persons who were privy to such information, but refused to disclose it."[11]

Disinformation has been another malicious quandary for the searchers and survivors. Unlike a lack of information, disinformation is cruelly deceitful. For example, through the end of the 1990s, most Bosniaks (at least 70 percent) believed that their missing family members were somewhere in Bosnia, in prisoner-of-war camps or "working as forced laborers in mines across the border in Serbia."[12] These rumors, many circulated by Bosnian Serbs, spread like wildfire in the Bosnian collection centers where survivors gathered daily for information about missing family, and led to irrational hopes that their missing son, husband, or father was still alive—somewhere.

On August 29, 2014,[13] for the first time since the wars ended in 1995, the presidents of the belligerent states, Bosnia, Croatia, and Serbia, signed a "landmark" declaration designed to speed up the search for "around 13,000 people whose bodies have not been found." The signing took place in Mostar, Bosnia, and was aimed at ending the *horrific crime*" of silence about the location of the still-unknown gravesites. Bakir Izetbegovic, the presiding member of the Bosnian tripartite presidency, said that while "we know we might never find all the victims, we will not give up while there is hope. This is why [we] are calling on those who have information about graves to cooperate with us. *It is the humane thing to do.*"[14] (my emphasis)

POLITICAL OBSTRUCTION. Some of the perpetrators "are still in important positions and are still very influential political figures. . . . Covering up these crimes is in their interest. Their logic is that if there are no bodies, there is no crime, and they won't be prosecuted," said Kathryne Bomberger, the ICMP's general director.[15]

Unfortunately, although all sides in the Bosnian war took actions that frustrated efforts to find the missing, the chief culprits are the Bosnian Serbs. They operated "with great arrogance," said one forensic anthropologist. "They didn't believe that anyone would actually come to the killing fields and look for these bodies after the fact. The wires were [even] left on people's wrists."[16]

In addition, before the forensic teams even began field-work, some "wily" Bosnian Serbs dug up and burned many corpses, loaded other dead bodies onto trucks and drove them from the gravesites to Serbia, or reburied them in secondary graves in the country. However, as Koff notes in her book, "the power of human remains puts the lie to government denial about the murder of civilians by their soldiers. To find three bodies, let alone more than 100 bodies of the Vukovar Hospital dead, is to lay waste to those claims."[17]

REBURIAL OF BODIES. A basic strategy of the Bosnian Serbs in their cover-up of the executed bodies was the constant reburial of the mortal remains of their victims. Repeatedly, backhoes and bulldozers were used to dig up the dead and move them to other locations to bar detection and criminal action against the killers by the ICTY and Bosnian prosecutors.

The killers plant the bones in newly dug graves, deposit them in the land's natural depressions, or drop the bodies in deep caves. They divide and place mortal remains in new mass graves in different locations, in order to conceal their crimes. One forensic professional angrily said: "Each time we open a grave we find a hand, a bone, or maybe even a head of a person we have found parts of before."[18]

In 1996, one such removal and reburial caught the attention of Bosnian searchers and reporters. A mass grave was found in a deep cave near the site of the Serb-run Omarska concentration camp in northwestern Bosnia. In the Serbs' attempt to conceal the crime, perpetrators threw bodies of dead animals and garbage on top of the human remains and set off an explosion in the cave.[19] Their clear goal was to prevent the searchers from finding the evidence of their brutal work.

They failed in that attempt but have, to date, succeeded in other efforts to conceal the evidence of their crimes— the human remains of their victims. "Nowhere else in the world has this occurred during time of war," wrote one scholar about the secondary mass graves tactic.[20]

SOME DANGERS CONFRONTING THE SEARCHERS. The major difference between the forensic scientist working in an American morgue to identify the cause of death and the forensic scientist at work in Bosnia is the "immersion in a military environment" the latter experiences. As William Haglund, one of the first Americans to work in Bosnia, said, "We wore flak jackets, we were under armed guard. This is a place where if the sign says 'Keep Off the Grass,' you keep off the grass because it's mined."[21]

In 1992 the UN Commission on Experts took its initial action to find physical evidence of war crimes and crimes against humanity. The organization requested the Physicians for Human Rights (PHR), an international NGO, to bring a forensic team into the Vukovar, Croatia, area to examine a suspicious rubbish dump. Earlier, the ICRC found evidence of criminal activities, including three surface skeletons of men with gunshot wounds to their heads. Clearly, the dump was a gravesite.

However, "the forensic team was run off the site at gunpoint by local Serbian authorities. The only solution was for the UN to protect the grave from tampering until a forensic team could return in safety. Soldiers ended up guarding the site for four years, until exhumation began again in 1996."[22]

The forensic scientists searching for the disappeared in Bosnia lived and worked in Republika Srpska territory because that area once was Muslim territory. It was in this soil that the Bosniaks went missing. The searchers had to work in fields occupied by Bosnian Serbs, men who, years earlier, probably killed the people the searchers were seeking.[23] The Serbs despised the forensics personnel for they could—and did—find damaging evidence of war crimes that led to indictments by the ICTY prosecutor's office.

The forensic personnel, therefore, lived in large tents at NATO's IFOR military bases. Each workday at a gravesite meant a drive of up to two hours to the evacuation area—accompanied by one hundred American IFOR troops who then protected the scientists at the gravesite. After working until dusk, the forensics team had to return to the base—with their IFOR escorts. Early on in the searching process, "they were in constant danger of being attacked by Serb paramilitaries."[24]

There was also the fear that the Bosnian Serbs, after the searchers left the excavation site in the evening, would damage, sabotage, or booby-trap the site. Since the IFOR commanders did not provide personnel to guard the sites, forensic scientists often slept there to prevent Serb actions that, if successful, would destroy evidence of war crimes.[25]

Further endangering the searchers' mission—and their

lives—was the reality of more than three million live land mines in the territory. Moreover, there were no maps showing the location of the mines. To travel the roads to the sites, demining sappers with their dogs had to clear the roads— and the sites themselves—of mines so that the forensics team could hike safely to a spot, work the gravesite, "and walk to a place to pee."[26]

This grim reality of all wars-—the unexploded mines— accounts for the deaths of many hundreds of military personnel since 1995 (more than four hundred military killed or wounded in the Croatian fields alone). In addition, there are the civilian deaths—people who were simply walking or playing in the countryside.

Clea Koff wrote about the fears the forensics personnel experienced because of the mines. Most of the mines planted by the Bosnian Serbs "were anti-personnel devices cleverly disguised as grass and dirt—they looked so much like what we work with when locating graves. The mines sat like little turds in the meadows."[27]

New Scientific Techniques for Finding the Missing

Amor Masovic, one of the directors of the MPI, has been searching for the missing for two decades. Some farmers, he said, "say that they can find these [graves] by searching for a special species of blue butterfly, but I rely on the scientific method."[28] Finding the missing graves in 2015 "is [still] the epitome of the proverbial needle in the haystack," said a Canadian researcher recently, working on a new technology to assist the searchers.[29] Given the obstacles facing Masovic and other grave-searchers, there have been a number of new scientific techniques developed to help find the missing graves.

By 2005 the organizations searching for the graves (the ICMP, PHR, and the MPI) were using them in earnest. Comparing satellite pictures taken in 1995 with the latest images enables the searchers to see vegetation patches that do not match the surrounding terrain. After noting the vegetative anomaly, an excavation team takes a closer look at the plants growing there.

Sites with human remains under the ground "are usually wetter than sites without" mortal remains. Running electricity into the ground measures the soil's resistance to the current. The possible gravesites "are less resistant to the electric current. [Once these are found] . . . the field team will then do a physical probe to check for remains."[30]

Using satellite imagery, vegetative analysis, and electrical resistivity technology has also enabled the searchers to locate the reburied secondary sites. Until these technological strategies became operational, searchers had to rely on the infrequent informant tip-off to them about the reburial locations.[31]

Another breakthrough came in 2005 when English and American scientists announced they had detected "geographic patterns associated with mass graves." These gravesites are "characteristically found in river valleys; in the corner of meadows or agricultural fields; within 100 meters of a road; on a low slope from the road to the site; and colonized by dense weeds and grasses."[32] Using these technological aids together enables the searchers to "find patterns and differences in the ground [they] know are associated with mass graves."[33]

Scientists know that a decomposing body under the ground can fertilize a plant for years and releases chemicals that stain the soil above the human remains.[34] In 2010 scientists working at McGill University in Montreal developed special cameras that measure changes in the light coming from soil and plants. The technology, hyperspectral imaging, is a type of "remote sensing."[35] The camera "collects and processes light from across the electromagnetic spectrum, including visible light, as well as ultraviolet and infrared light." If there is any decay under the ground, up to eight feet deep, the searcher can see a difference. "After five years, plants growing over buried bodies suddenly reflect light instead of absorbing light. In fact, on-grave plants reflect more than twice the green light of off-grave plants. For a human eye, detecting such tiny changes would be very hard, but the difference is obvious to the hyperspectral camera."[36]

These new technological devices are of immense help to the ICMP and MPI forensic teams in the Bosnian fields. However, in the end, only on-site archeological excavation and exhumation confirms these scientific findings.

Phase Two: Site Excavation and Evidence Recovery

Under international humanitarian law, diggings and exhumations are the responsibility of the former belligerents.[37] However, the UN and major humanitarian organizations have taken over this primary task in Bosnia and other killing fields. It is critically important that a suspected gravesite be located and the exhumation process conducted by forensic professionals, especially forensic anthropologists.

The gravesite is *always* approached with great care because of the possibility that it is mined or layered with unexploded ordnance. Military deminers are the professionals who handle the dangerous problem. Forensic specialists with the ICMP, the PHR, and the MPI are the major participants in the excavation and evidence recovery phase after demining ends. In addition, present at every exhumation are representatives from Bosnia's prosecutor's office, a medical expert, and police.

After military personnel or special professional demining teams remove mines and other dangerous ordnance, the exhumation process begins. The recovery team starts by very carefully probing the grave, using metal rods, "seeking to test its consistency and detect the smell of dead bodies. Once investigators have dug down to the level of bodies, they will sift the earth for shreds of evidence and dust off each body. Bodies are carefully examined before being removed. Valuable evidence can include blindfolds, bullets, and bonds that will indicate how a victim was killed. Jewelry or papers help with identification."[38]

The field investigators document information about the site. Photographs are taken of the human and other remains found in the grave for subsequent identification and possible criminal indictments in the ICTY and Bosnia's criminal courts. (Since 2011 the Bosnian Prosecutor's Office is in overall charge of every exhumation because "all graves are considered to be possible crime scenes." A prosecutor must be present at the excavation site for any evidence to be admissible in court.[39])

The exhumation of the gravesite can take days or months, depending on the size and its complexity, the terrain, the remoteness of the site, and the danger of mines in the site itself and in the roads leading to it. All the mortal remains from the site, carefully bagged, are taken to the closest of a dozen mortuary facilities, called Identification Coordination Centers, in Bosnia and placed in cold storage. It is at these locations that the laborious and frustrating identification process begins.[40]

The Third Phase: Identification of the Victim and Cause of Death in the Mortuary

Finding the graves can take many decades and, unfortunately, not all of the missing are found. Once mortal remains arrive at the mortuary facility, professional investigators—pathologists, radiologists, forensic anthropologists, photographers, cultural anthropologists, odontologists, data entry staff, and support team members (engineers, drivers, technicians, mechanics) "carry out detailed pathological, anthropological, radiographic, forensic, and investigative analysis to assist in judicial and humanitarian identifications."[41]

The mortuary itself must be in a secure location, in close proximity to both the field sites and the forensic team's home base. At a minimum, the facility must be located in a large open area, with sufficient electric and water, air conditioning, refrigeration, and heat. The mortuary must have a variety of rooms for different needs associated with investigating the cause and manner of death of the victims.

There must be, for example, separate dressing areas for the forensics team, sanitation facilities, a refrigerated holding area for the mortal remains, the body processing room (autopsy tables), a waiting room for relatives to view bodies, staff rest areas, an equipment room, a postmortem examination room, and a refrigerated storage area for human remains after postmortem examination.[42]

In the mortuary, the bones are placed on worktables, cleaned, and "laid out in anatomical position for examination. [Forensic pathologists] retain the following samples for eventual DNA analysis: mid-shaft of the femur or humerus . . . and premolar and/or molar tooth."[43] Other support technicians clean clothing found on or near the bones in the mortuary's clothes-washing room.

The primary reason for the extensive delay in identifying many remains is the already-noted Serb tactic of movement of body parts—often more than twice. It is a common cause of identification delay because body parts are scattered in many graves. Hazreta Mustafic, wife of a missing person, lost all her male relatives during the war. "My uncle's body was found in seven separate locations," she told a reporter in 2011.[44]

Furthermore, until the forensic teams began to use DNA evidence to identify the bones in November 2001, the identification process of "unknown remains was extremely slow because of a lack of documents [personal information about a missing person, e.g., broken bones, x-rays], distinctive clothing or personal belongings."[45] Prior to the use of DNA technology in 2001, identification of the mortal remains rarely occurred. Family members of missing persons viewed a book of photographs (clothing, watches, jewelry, shoes) prepared by the ICRC in the hope that they could identify an object that belonged to the missing person. (Since passage of the Bosnian Law on Missing Persons in 2004, the status of a missing person changes *only* when the mortal remains are identified.[46])

In 2015 the primary method for identifying the remains is the scientific one: the DNA process. However, the traditional method is still used by ICRC and ICMP staff. For example, there are days when clothing and artifacts found in the mass graves are laid out in front of the mortuary so that surviving family members can view and touch the articles to see if any belonged to their disappeared son, husband, or father.

Traditional or Classical Method

This identification of human remains technique is based on the collection of information about the missing person from interactions between the ICRC, the PHR, and ICMP staff with the missing person's family members. The victim's identity could be determined in part by identification of his clothes, personal belongings, or documents found in the grave. In addition, ICRC, PHR, and ICMP personnel collect *antemortem*[47] *data* (AMD) from interviews with surviving family members. Antemortem data is information about the missing person while he/she was alive. It "can be dental x-rays, old fractures that have been x-rayed, medical histories that show diseases in the bone that might be apparent [in the mortuary], and basic things like age, sex, stature, left handed and right handedness, all these things point you to who this individual was."[48]

Each person's physical characteristics are unique. Using AMD with information collected during autopsy examination, the forensic scientists attempt to identify the human remains. In the early years of the identification process, there were few antemortem records. With the development of a basic antemortem database protocol by Laurie Vollen in 1997, a public health doctor with PHR, the interview process quickly emerged and the AMD database grew exponentially.[49]

The antemortem database's purpose is to help forensic staff identify large numbers of human remains. PHR and ICRC staff interviewed thousands of survivors to gather all possible identifying information on the missing and put the information in one searchable computer record. The data is matched up with physical evidence from the mortal remains to try to identify the body.[50]

An unusual AMD surfaced after the Srebrenica killings. Because the town was under Bosnian Serb military occupation for three years, there was no way to buy new clothing. The women who survived used "their memories of their own sewing" to identify the clothing pulled out of the grave. During the long siege, the wives and mothers constantly made repairs to their husband's or son's clothing. And they used distinctive stitching patterns that, years later, were identified by many of the women.[51]

However, regrettably, using these traditional techniques between 1996 and 2001, "only a few more than 100 people were identified."[52] Only after the ICMP forensic scientists introduced the DNA technology did the identification process show great success in identifying the victims. By 2003, using DNA data, "the ICMP has been instrumental in closing over 1,000 missing person cases. . . . DNA matching has drastically expedited the identification process."[53]

Scientific Method: Use of DNA *Extraction to*
Identify the Human Remains

For the forensic scientists working for PHR and ICMP, the "forensic revolution [that began in 2001] is that we *begin* the identification process with the DNA. With computers we compare the DNA profiles of the remains against the DNA profiles of the families to generate cold matches," said Adnan Rizvic, in 2003 the head of the ICMP's Identification Coordination Program.[54]

The bone-blood DNA matching system innovated in Bosnia was unique in forensic science. Created in 1999 by Ed Huffine, an American forensic geneticist, the new technique "stood conventional DNA on its head. Conventional DNA analysis *confirmed* or *excluded* an already presumed link or identification. In Bosnia, DNA analysis was the *matching* of genetic profiles; it acted as the engine for the entire identification process."[55]

To use the new DNA methodology, it is "vital" that the forensic scientists have sufficient family blood reference samples that will be compared to the DNA remains recovered from the bones of the victim. By 2011, "there were more than 90,000 relatives' blood samples ready to be matched" with victim DNA.[56]

Optimally, a DNA profile from the bones of the victim is paired with DNA from family members. In the major mortuary facility, located in Tuzla, called by forensic specialists the "body factory,"[57] there is a blood analysis facility with technological equipment to extract DNA samples from the bones. The bone's surface "is cleaned of flesh and dirt, the bone marrow is bleached, it is ground down, [sent to a laboratory in Sarajevo, where the sample is powdered and] the DNA extract taken from that," said senior ICMP scientist Jon Davoren.[58]

For confirmation purposes using DNA, the match must be *minimally* 99.95 percent certain. In almost all matches, the level of certainty is 100 percent.[59] However, identification of all victims is not possible. There may be no family reference samples for a DNA comparison. Many surviving family members emigrated to Europe or North America; they are not able to provide their DNA for comparison. Many times, *entire* families disappeared in the war. Sometimes there is no intact DNA extracted from the mortal remains.

If there is a DNA match, a report is prepared and sent to the MPI. That organization forwards the report to the court-appointed medical expert and the prosecutor's office. Their task is to consider all the evidence, including AMD, to confirm the DNA match. The medical expert must also file an opinion on the possible cause of death that the prosecutor will review for possible future legal action.

If there is confirmation of the report, then a municipal registrar's office person issues a death certificate.[60] The surviving family members receive the remains of their now-found missing victim. Burial follows, which is a crucial religious and communal custom for Bosniaks.

"Now I know where his grave is," said a survivor about his dead brother. "I know this is the end of the story. Before there was a little bit of hope. We thought he might still be alive and might appear one day. But now the story has ended. The uncertainty has ended."[61] For others, while the uncertainty ends, "one chapter ends, another one starts. We have reached the truth. Now we want to see justice being done."[62]

For many survivors, the science of DNA was bewildering, unfathomable. "They were skeptical and confused about genetic testing,"[63] and it took patience and education by ICRC and ICMP staff to overcome the lack of understanding and the distrust the survivors held about the process.

For some women whose men were missing, the work of the forensic investigators angered them. "They were sure that their men were alive, in POW camps in Serbia, and political pressure—not excavation of rubbish pits—was what was needed to bring them home."[64]

Koff was shocked when a delegation of the women demonstrated against her forensic team in 1996. They were not happy to see the workers "arrive with a bunch of shovels."[65] Koff wrote, *"They didn't want to be survivors of the dead, but rather seekers of the living.* The relatives didn't want anything back from us because to get anything is to acknowledge that their loved ones are dead."[66] (my emphasis)

In a way, all surviving family members secretly shared this attitude of the Vukovar women, however unrealistic it was. Most of the women across Bosnia, however, did not angrily confront the forensic scientists.

From "Grave to Grave": Summarizing the Identification Process

In Bosnia DNA identity testing is primarily conducted by the ICMP. Each forensic team generally has sixteen members.[67] There are two forensic anthropology teams in the group. One does the mapping of the site, logging data, photographing the bodies, and wrapping the hands in a plastic bag, along with any clothing found by the remains. The second team then exhumes the body, places it in a numbered body bag, places the body on a stretcher and carries the remains to a refrigerated container for transport to the nearest morgue.

The forensic specialists in Bosnia and all other postconflict work areas follow a standard protocol created by the ICMP for identifying the victims:

1. Demarcate the area in which the forensic anthropologist found the remains.

2. A piece of paper with the reference code for the body is placed with the remains.

3. The remains are photographed.

4. The individual exhumation site is dismantled as body parts are put in a plastic bag.

5. The bones are brought to a reassociation center for possible reassociation of bones—upper body with lower body, skulls with torsos.

6. Forensic anthropologists carefully examine each of the bones one at a time to narrow the field of subsequent DNA testing.

7. The remains are moved to the mortuary facility in Tuzla or one of the other facilities throughout the nation. There is further cleaning of the remains and separation of clothing from the remains; they are washed and placed in paper bags with the same reference number on them.

8. The forensic pathologist, with assistance from forensic anthropologists, observed by police and prosecutor's office representatives, begins the autopsy examination.

9. Bone samples or a tooth are sent to the bone department for further cleaning and cataloging.

10. Artifacts (watches, eyeglasses, religious medallions, jewelry) are collected, cleaned, and numbered by a Forensic Evidence technician.

11. The samples receive a bar code before being transferred to Sarajevo for DNA extraction and analysis.

12. There the technicians extract DNA from each sample, producing a *genetic profile* by reading the sixteen sites

found along the DNA strand—this profile is the analysis's most valuable and powerful tool.

13. The numbers in the profile are fed into the computer software program, which searches through nearly one hundred thousand samples of blood taken by surviving family members in order to find their match—"to reunite the missing person with his genetic kin." In addition, the technicians carefully screen the profiles and the AMD collected from surviving family members; it is a "kind of genetic detective work" to assess the probability that the two profiles match.

14. To have a match the statistics have to be good, that is, they have to pass the 99.95 percent threshold for the match to advance the case into the final stages of identification.

15. After there has been a positive match, the results are forwarded to the MPI, which then sends the documents to the court-appointed medical officer and prosecutor, who make sure all the examinations are complete and that the evidence confirms the DNA match. The medical officer's opinion on the cause of death is sent to the prosecutor's office.

16. Death confirmation is sent to the municipal registrar's office, and that office issues a death certificate.

17. Finally, ICMP and ICRC staff visit with the surviving family members to tell them of the results of the process and arrange for the transportation of the mortal remains to them for burial.[68]

As Wagner writes, "the identification of mortal remains presents the single abiding resolution to this [emotional dilemma]. It bridges the enormous and dreadful chasm between surviving family members' memories of the missing and their imaginings about the nature of their relatives' death and the place of their bones."[69]

The Major Organizations Working to Find and Identify the Disappeared in Bosnia

After the Dayton Peace Accords took effect on December 14, 1995, tracing the disappeared in Bosnia-Herzegovina "became a joint effort of the parties [Serbia, Bosnia, Croatia, Republika Srpska] and various international organizations."[70] Each former warring party established a Government Commission for Detained and Missing Persons. IFOR and then SFOR military forces, most from NATO nations, were tasked with the protection of forensic specialists working to find missing gravesites. The UN's High Commissioner for Refugees (UNHCR) is the international agency responsible— with the assistance of the ICRC—for assisting the tens of thousands of internally displaced families in Bosnia and Croatia.

The Accords stipulated that the ICRC was to assure that "all tracing requests and information concerning missing persons shall be transmitted to the Central Tracing Agency of the ICRC." Further, the ICRC "reversed its policy regarding the evacuation of mass graves and indicated its interest in getting directly involved in exhumation activities. As a result, the ICRC assumed the long term custody of the ante-mortem database."[71]

Another nongovernmental organization (NGO), Physicians for Human Rights (PHR), appeared in the 1997 UN Report. The organization "entered into a collaborative relationship with the ICTY and started in July 1996 to exhume mass graves in Bosnia and Croatia on behalf of the Tribunal. In addition to providing evidence for ICTY, the autopsies also lead to the identification of deceased missing persons." In addition, it had "overall responsibility for the establishment and maintenance of the AMD, including the development of a computer database, the overall methodology of the project, and a comprehensive questionnaire of all pertinent information regarding missing persons which is necessary for the purpose of identification by comparing it to post-mortem information recovered at the time of autopsy of victims exhumed from mass graves. This information includes physical characteristics, type of clothing worn, personal effects, and history of injuries and damage to bones and teeth."[72]

Forensic teams from Finland, Austria, and the Netherlands supported the UN in its exhumation efforts. The Finnish team, the Finnish Civil-Military Cooperation Center (CIMIC), is still working in the country on a number of tasks, including helping refugees, demining, and providing security for the forensic teams. These teams are part of the Joint Forensic Expert Commission on Exhumation. On October 11, 1997, another key group came into being: the International Commission on Missing Persons (ICMP).

What these forensics institutions brought to the Balkan region was the expertise and knowledge needed to deal with the task of finding and identifying the missing. The ICMP and PHR brought the experts who developed and implemented cutting-edge techniques vital to the task.

For example, a team of Scottish forensic pathologists arrived in 1996 to set up and staff the major mortuary in Tuzla. It was urgently needed because the conflict ended and the mortal remains were being found and readied for further forensic work. Robert McNeil, the NHS Glasgow mortuaries operations manager, headed the team that set up the mortuary. Kerry-Ann Martin, a forensic anthropologist from Wales, came to work in it.[73]

Another example of the introduction of external assistance was the knowledge brought to the field in 2001 by a forensic geneticist from the United States, John Crews.

The ICMP asked Crews, chief of forensic genetics and laboratory director of the NGO Guatemala Forensic Anthropology Foundation (GFAT), to implement the DNA identification program created by Huffine in 1999 because Bosnia "had almost no DNA capability." After Crews finished his work establishing the first DNA laboratory, the victim identification rate was pushed to 80 percent, which was, as already noted, "unprecedented."[74]

In the years since the Dayton Peace Accords took effect, four organizations have continued the burdensome task of finding, exhuming, and identifying the disappeared in Bosnia: the ICRC, ICMP, PHR, and the Bosnian government agency named, since 2005, the Missing Persons Institute (MPI).

International Committee of the Red Cross (ICRC)

The ICRC is the oldest international humanitarian organization. In 1859 a Swiss citizen from Geneva, Henri Dunant, helped wounded soldiers at the battle of Solverino. Afterward he pushed nations to do more to provide medical and humanitarian work to protect war victims—soldiers and civilians alike. In 1863 he created the ICRC. It began with two goals on its agenda: writing and implementing a treaty[75] that would provide wounded and captured soldiers with medical and civilized care, and creating national Red Cross human relief associations.[76] Its mission statement lays out the broad parameters of the ICRC:

> The ICRC is an impartial, neutral, and independent organization whose exclusively humanitarian mission is to protect the lives and dignity of victims of armed conflict and other situations of violence and to provide them with assistance. The ICRC also endeavors to prevent suffering by promoting and strengthening humanitarian law and humanitarian principles.... It directs and coordinates the international activities

conducted by the Movement in armed conflicts and other situations of violence.[77]

The ICRC's work, in the twenty-first century, remains twofold: operational, "helping victims of armed conflict and other situations of violence and developing and promoting humanitarian law and humanitarian principles."[78] In Bosnia, the ICRC's goal is to help find missing persons and work with the former warring parties to implement international humanitarian law, especially with respect to the many problems refugees face.

The ICRC's view is that, "in war, many people go missing, causing anguish and uncertainty for their families and friends. People have the right to know what happened to their missing relatives. Government, the military authorities, and armed groups have an obligation to provide information and assist efforts to put families back together."[79]

For ICRC leaders, this issue was a global "hidden tragedy" that had to be addressed by the world community. It did not attract "sufficient attention" from the nations and, in 2003, the ICRC organized an international conference on finding the missing and helping the families of the disappeared.

Since 1996 the ICRC is at work in the western Balkans; there is a delegation and working group located in Belgrade, Serbia (covering Albania, Croatia, Macedonia, Montenegro, and Serbia). Another delegation is located in Sarajevo. The ICRC's main role is to support efforts to determine the fate of missing people "and to ensure that their families' legal, psychological, and economic needs are met."[80]

The Dayton Peace Accords called for the ICRC to "clarify the fate of all persons remaining unaccounted for. The work of the ICRC is focused on endeavors to secure the cooperation of authorities in locating and identifying missing persons and support their families."[81]

In 2002 an article appeared in the ICRC's publication

FINDING, EXHUMING, AND IDENTIFYING REMAINS

addressing some problems faced by the ICRC when implementing this mandate.[82] "Should a humanitarian organization like the ICRC destroy hope when it is often impossible to be absolutely certain that a missing person is dead? May the ICRC conversely perpetuate suffering, if only by omission, simply because absolute certainty does not exist? Should the ICRC leave it to the families to decide what they want?"[83]

In an attempt to answer these questions, the ICRC initially resorted to the issuance of death certificates based on AMD about a missing relative and confirmation of the person's death "by the relevant authorities on the other side."[84] After double-checking the data, if the ICRC representative is satisfied that the person was deceased, a "Certificate of Death" was issued and delivered to the family.

However, the program "caused a backlash; many, though not all, refused to accept a 'paper death,' as long as the body was not returned. They also believed that this kind of information was meant to make them stop searching."[85]

In the fall of 1997, the death certificate program ended. The Bosniaks "were unwilling or unable to accept an ICRC 'paper death.'" An ICRC worker explained this response: "Without a body or, at least, a photograph of a corpse or a piece of clothing," the missing family member was not dead.[86]

The ICRC's mission is to save lives, protect and assist living people, and enable families to be reunited. However, the ICRC now works "on the assumption that a missing person is alive and detained."[87] The consequences are clear: the survivors' hopes are confirmed and the mourning process is delayed.

International Commission on Missing Persons (ICMP)

The major NGO involved in finding the disappeared is the International Commission on Missing Persons (ICMP). Established at the urging of President Bill Clinton in 1996 at the G-7 Summit in Lyon, France, the primary role of the ICMP, then and now, is to "ensure the cooperation of [former enemy] governments in locating and identifying those who have disappeared during armed conflict or as a result of human rights violations."[88]

> When it began work in 1997, the ICMP had 20 professionals working in Bosnia. In 2011, with 170 forensic specialists working across the world [in twenty-seven countries], it is the largest investigative forensic organization in existence. It is organized into four main areas: the forensic program, family association development, the political program, and the DNA program (which includes the training of specialists to do DNA analysis).
>
> Its funding comes from less than two dozen nations. The United States is the major contributor to the organization. The major tool for identifying the mortal remains is DNA. In 2001, before its use, there were only 52 remains identified. One year later, after DNA began to be used, the number of identified remains stood at 518—ten times greater than the previous year.[89]

President Clinton said that the primary tasks of the new organization were "to secure the *full cooperation of all the parties* to the Dayton peace agreement in locating the missing from the four year conflict and to assist them in doing so . . . to support and enhance the work of other organizations in their efforts to encourage public involvement in its activities and to contribute to the development of appropriate expressions of commemoration and tribute to the missing."[90] (my emphasis)

Getting the former warring entities to work together to locate, exhume, and identify the missing in the Bosnian war was and remains a troublesome problem because of the hatred spewed during and after the conflict. ICMP staff has to address the bitterness and distrust existing between Croats, Bosniaks, and Serbs to overcome the existing political inertia of these entities. As former ICMP chairman Cyrus Vance said in 1997, "Politically, we have pressed the parties to intensify their cooperation in the exhumation and identification process, and to release all their forensic and other records about the missing. [However,] I remain disappointed by the lack of cooperation between the parties in expediting the process of exhumation and identification. . . . The ICMP needs to focus more on this vital issue."[91]

In 2015, however, the tension remains between the entities. It is seen in Bosnia's hostile reaction to the arrests of Muslim men suspected of abducting, torturing, and killing Bosnian Serb and Croat citizens living in the Sarajevo area during the three-year siege of Sarajevo and "shows that the culture of denial embraces all sides in Bosnia."[92]

Working toward resolving the "vital issue," the ICMP is engaged in the development and support of local associations of families of missing persons. Working with other NGOs in the area of human rights, more than 120 associations now function in Croatia, Bosnia, and Serbia.[93]

Working with the ICRC on the Ante-Mortem Database Project, the ICMP, by the end of 2008, developed a database of ninety thousand relatives of some thirty thousand missing people. More than thirty-three thousand DNA samples from mortal remains exhumed from the mass graves have enabled the ICMP, in its Identification Coordination Centers, to identify nearly sixteen thousand people who were tagged as missing by their family members. The DNA identification success rate since 2008 has increased substantially. This encouraging fact reflects the arduous work of the ICMP to get the three groups to work more cooperatively in finding the mass graves, exhuming them, and getting the mortal remains to the mortuaries located across the traumatized nation.

Since 2001, given the success of the organization's use of DNA technology in mass identifications, the ICMP "has been transformed from a small institution operating on an essentially political level into the biggest identification program in the world. ICMP currently operates the world's largest high-throughput screening DNA human identification facility."[94]

The ICMP is now a worldwide organization that uses its expertise to help other nations locate and identify missing persons after natural disasters and when hostilities end. It provides technical assistance, including DNA analysis and forensic specialists. Currently, the main office of the ICMP is located in Sarajevo. (It will be relocated to The Hague in 2015.) However, it has assisted governments in the Middle East, Latin America, Southeast Asia, and the United States (after Hurricane Katrina devastated Louisiana). In addition, the ICMP, unlike the neutral ICRC, "responds to requests for documentation and expert reports from international and domestic courts on matters related to war crimes, crimes against humanity, genocide, and other crimes under international law."[95]

Repeatedly, the ICMP informs the public in Croatia, Bosnia, and Serbia of one major remaining problem: the lack of information about the undiscovered mass graves.

> We constantly appeal to the public to inform us or the MPI— they can do this anonymously—about any location they suspect may hide an individual or mass burial site, or about a crime that took place and bodies were hidden.

> . . . We don't have the mandate for criminal prosecution or war crimes. That is a job for other institutions. What we want is to find these people, return them to their families, and to allow the survivors to have some semblance of normal life in the future.[96]

As one ICMP staff person put it, the organization's essential goal "is to provide the family with as much of their loved ones as possible."[97]

Physicians for Human Rights (PHR)

Carola Eisenberg, a teenager in 1930s Argentina, visited a psychiatric hospital. There she saw thirty-five hundred patients chained to beds. This exposure to such inhumane treatment led her to fight for humane health care and, in 1986, to found the NGO, Physicians for Human Rights (PHR), in Cambridge, Massachusetts.[98]

The five founders of PHR focused on efforts to alleviate suffering across the globe. In 1997 the PHR shared the Nobel Prize for Peace. By 2011 PHR's medical and forensic specialists worked in more than forty countries, including Iraq and Cyprus. Since it began operations in 1986, "PHR has sent more than [one hundred] medical and forensic teams to dozens of countries to carry out forensic investigations, including exhumations and autopsies of deceased victims of alleged torture and extrajudicial executions."[99] The doctors who founded the NGO shared the same commitment to alleviate suffering that Eisenberg expressed: "their training as physicians and the ethical commitments that accompany their profession demand that they identify transgressions and offer a voice to the powerless."[100]

One, Dr. Jonathan Fine, had a similar experience that Eisenberg had in the 1930s. He visited Chile while General Augusto Pinochet was the dictatorial leader to meet with imprisoned Chilean doctors. Their jailers had psychologically tortured the Chileans. "He was stunned by what he saw and heard, and although the physicians were released 5 weeks after his visit, Fine was spurred to action."[101]

The commitment of PHR was clear from the very beginning: to use the scientific expertise and authority of medical professionals to bring human rights violations to light and provide justice for victims. The PHR mission statement says clearly, "PHR exists to stop mass atrocities (crimes against humanity, genocide, and war crimes) and acts that cause severe physical or mental harm to individuals."[102]

After the Dayton Peace Accords, in 1996 the PHR began its work by exhuming mass graves. This activity is one of the primary actions of the group: investigating abuses using forensic science, from exhumation to the use of DNA in autopsies and identification of the victims. The organization's forensic scientists have been working at the ICTY at The Hague to produce evidence of war crimes for the court. Their documenting of evidence in autopsy work is prepared for possible legal action by criminal tribunals and commissions.

The organization created the International Forensics Program (IFP) in 1987. Forensic specialists—all volunteers—working for PHR include forensic anthropologists and pathologists, and experts from other analytical sciences in forensics labs. It is "dedicated to providing independent forensic expertise to document and collect evidence of human rights violations or violations of international humanitarian law."[103]

An important facet of the IFP is the forensic training the PHR provides to human rights workers and investigators of interested nations so that they can work on this activity in the future. The courses, taught online and annually at the PHR's Cambridge, Massachusetts, headquarters, include forensic science, crime scenes and evidence documentation, human identification, DNA analysis, and international forensic examinations. Customized training can be provided "on a case-specific basis to human rights organizations and their investigators."[104]

The Bosnia Missing Persons Institute (MPI)

Another important development in the hunt to find and identify the missing occurred in 1998. Until then, the two very autonomous "entities" in Bosnia, the Federation of

Bosnia-Herzegovina (Muslims and Croats) and the Republika Srpska, had their own missing persons organizations and did not share information and data with each other.[105] "There has been a power struggle as regards information. The Serbian victims get no information from the Federation and the Republika Srpska gives little information back. We are talking about both mistrust and downright obstruction. The local commissions for missing persons have always just excavated 'their own.' The one commission—in the Bosnian-Croat Federation—has searched for Bosnian Croats and Bosniaks, while the second commission—in the Republika Srpska—has searched for Bosnian Serbs. This means that the commissions for all these years since peace was declared [in 1995], have contributed to a polarization and distrust between the groups."[106]

The peacemakers, especially the leaders of the ICRC and the ICMP, aware of this reality, introduced a proposal in 1998 to create a Missing Persons Institute for the recently created (1995) nation of Bosnia-Herzegovina that envisioned joint exhumation projects by the three former warring ethnic groups. Coordination and completion of the process became the task of the ICMP. This operation began in 2000 and the three entities conducted exhumations on the "opposing side's" territory to find "their" disappeared.

By 2003 "the political climate had become more conducive to the creation of joint institutions." Therefore, in the spring of 2003, ICMP believed it was time to go from entity-level to state-level work on finding the disappeared. ICMP leaders met with the tripartite presidency "and invited Bosnia to become a co-founder of the MPI along with the ICMP."

There was unanimous consent, and work began on the creation of the protocols for the new state institution. Involved in the process were the Council of Ministers (representing Bosnia), the ICMP, the ICRC, government officials, and associations of families of missing persons.

In August 2005, after two years of consulting and bargaining between the parties, an agreement was signed. In 2006 the first three members of the Board of Directors took their posts; in the summer of 2007 members of the bureaucracy came aboard. Finally, thirteen years after Dayton, in 2008, the MPI began its joint work. An ICMP spokesperson said: "The implementation of the MPI marks a milestone in the history of Bosnia and ICMP and provides a model for transitional justice that can be applied in many other situations and areas of the world. . . . This is no small feat."[107] Its purpose is clear: to provide the country "with a sustainable national mechanism to address the issue of persons missing as a result of the conflict, regardless of their ethnic, religious, or national origin." The MPI must also ensure that all mass and individual graves "are protected, catalogued, and properly evacuated."[108]

To that end, the first task of the MPI was the establishment of a unified record, the Central Records, of the missing on all sides of the Bosnian war. All the information previously collected by entity organizations—the ICMP, the ICRC, the PHR, and all other organizations—will be included in the Central Records of the MPI.

From its inception as an idea, the hope was that the MPI "will ultimately establish a central, transparent list of persons missing from the conflict in this country, which will leave no room for the damaging political manipulation of the numbers of victims that we have seen," said the director-general of the ICMP in August 2005 when the MPA was formally approved.[109] As will be seen in chapter 5, the ethnic enmity has not yet been replaced by cooperation. This continuing reality has adversely affected the success of the MPI.

Chapter 4 focuses on the day-to-day work of the mostly young forensic scientists, especially the forensic anthropologists, in the effort to find, exhume, and identify the disappeared in Bosnia.

FOUR

The Forensic Scientists at Work in Bosnia's "Killing Fields"

> Without knowledge of the whereabouts of their loved
> ones, there is always the hope, no matter how remote
> or irrational, that someday, somehow [the disappeared]
> may return. Through the efforts of the forensic scien-
> tists, relatives can be helped toward understanding and
> finally accepting the truth.
>
> —RICHARD GOLDSTONE

Forensic science "is the application of a science in a legal context."[1] It also is a collective term. The "reality is that there is no such individual as a 'forensic scientist.' The term denotes a class or group of areas spanning medicine, science, and technical fields."[2] The specific makeup of a forensic field team is determined by the availability of specialists, the resources available, the task to be performed, and the location of the site.

1992: The UN's Initial (Failed) Effort to Have Forensic Scientists Work in Bosnia

The ICTY was established by the UN in 1993. In part, its creation came about because the UN, months earlier, put together a forensic science field team, with the cooperation of the PHR, to examine the mortal remains of victims of a massacre at Vukovar, Croatia, when the JNA captured the city in 1992. The forensic team was instructed by the UN "to look into allegations of the removal of approximately two hundred patients and staff from the Vukovar Hospital. At the time it fell to the Serbs, there was a possible gravesite outside of town, at a place called Ovcara."[3] The group discovered many dead Croatian civilians in the mass graves and, after being sent out of the country by Serb authorities, filed their report with the UN.

Very quickly, because of these findings and the growing pressure to do *something* to address the horrors of the Bosnian wars, political actions in the UN led to the creation of the ICTY. Its charge: identify and prosecute the planners and organizers of genocide, war crimes, and crimes against humanity.[4] However, it took a number of years to staff the judges, the bureaucracy, and the prosecutor's office. When, in December 1995, the Dayton Peace Accords ended the wars, the Prosecutor's Office of the ICTY was ready to begin the task of bringing to trial the perpetrators of these crimes. The ICTY prosecutor, like any criminal prosecutor, needed hard evidence to indict and convict the persons responsible for ordering and implementing the crimes. He needed proof that the enemy had executed noncombatants during the war years. Such action taken by political leaders and their military forces is a violation of international humanitarian law, and the perpetrators are subject to indictment, trial, and conviction.

The mandate of the forensic teams in Bosnia followed from the ICTY's *raison d'être*: find the bodies, determine how they died, and send the evidence to The Hague for use by the ICTY prosecutor in criminal trials. The forensic teams were the only people who could provide the evidence needed by the prosecutor. In Bosnia, they succeeded in the awful task. As will be seen in this chapter, success came with heartrending sadness, nightmares, sleepless nights, and, at bottom, the knowledge that their work brought home to many survivors their missing husbands, sons, mothers, and fathers.

The Clash between the Humanitarian Needs of Families of the Missing and the Evidentiary Needs of the ICTY Prosecutors—with Forensic Scientists in the Middle

Justice Goldstone's comment about the value of the forensic scientists is somewhat perplexing because of the state of affairs in the late 1990s. In Bosnia and Rwanda, where war crimes and genocide occurred earlier in the decade, "identification of the victims was given *lower priority* than evidence collection, description of injuries, and cause of death determination."[5] (my emphasis)

The primary role of the special war crimes tribunals created by the UN, the ICTY in 1993 and the ICTR a year later, is to bring before the international criminal courts the alleged perpetrators of these crimes. The Office of the Prosecutor (OTP) contracted with forensic organizations such as PHR and, after 1997, the ICMP to send teams of forensic scientists to find the graves and to investigate the large-scale killings.

In July 1999, the OTP deputy prosecutor Graham Blewitt explained the needs—and the limitations—of the office. Because indictments are based on "circumstantial evidence, proving patterns is important. . . . We don't have to prove every single murder, or every single massacre, we just need to collect a sample of these so that we can prove a pattern of killing and destruction aimed against civilians."[6]

The underlying problem for the OTP is that the office in this period of time, "largely lack[ed] the resources . . . to undertake forensic investigations aimed at identifying *all* of the dead. . . . Personal identification of the victims may not be a necessary part of a *legal* investigation."[7]

In these early investigations, the forensic teams were requested by the ICTY to locate the graves; determine who was in the graves, that is, how many men, women, and children; find out how they were killed; and learn whether they were noncombatants—but not to ascertain the identity of a dead person. While there is, theoretically, a symbiotic relationship between the families of the missing and the goals of the prosecutor's office, the reality is that it did not then exist.[8]

As one forensic anthropologist said, "a tribunal is not particularly interested in individual identifications. They are interested in categorical identifications that would help them with their strategy in proving and showing lines of command and larger strategies. So in former Yugoslavia, if you prove that a grave had Muslims versus Croats versus Orthodox, or they were non-combatants versus combatants, or if they were bound or incapacitated in some way, that's a level of identification called categorical."[9]

The *primary* role of the forensic specialists working for the ICTY prosecutor's office is the *investigation* of the *cause of death* of recovered human remains. When they determine that deaths occurred with bullets, machetes, or strangulation, and that victims' hands were tied with wire and they were blindfolded, the data will be given to a state or international prosecutor's office for its evidentiary use in the criminal justice system. The forensic specialists' *secondary role*, the humanitarian one, is to try to uncover the identity of the mortal remains of the victim, regardless of the cause of death.

This placed the forensic specialists in an ethical quandary: does the team provide *only* the requisite evidence for the prosecutor, or do they continue to work to meet the needs of the families of the missing? Haglund answered this question in a way that all forensic scientists and staff accept: "If you lose sight that these graves contain individuals, then I think you should not be doing the work. Because the basic human right to me, and some people call it humanitarian desire and need, is that the families know the fate [of their family member]. Otherwise, they live in desperation with that question mark in their mind."[10]

As will be shown in this chapter, all forensic investigators work endlessly to *identify* the mortal remains. As one forensic anthropologist, who opted to finish all the exhumations, said: "It would have been disrespectful to leave."[11] All the forensic scientists feel this way about their work. Haglund, an experienced American forensic anthropologist, "said 'I always wore a suit and tie during my forensic work, in part out of my respect for the dead.'"[12] The forensic professionals were the advocates for the dead. They all wanted to right the wrongs they uncovered in their work. Haglund recalled the incident shortly after his arrival in Bosnia that framed his mindset: "I went into the cold room . . . and there was a child there, maybe about a six-year old child. And I pulled the sheet back and I saw a big boot imprint on his chest and a mark on his forehead, which we later determined to be a ring. And I thought, that child was helpless and innocent, and, really, we're their advocates. We speak for them. We are witnesses for them."[13]

By the early years of the twenty-first century, new funding allowed the ICMP to expand its staff of forensic specialists. Other NGOs, including PHR, the EAAF, and forensic teams from Guatemala, Norway, and Finland, increased the number of forensic staff in Bosnia. As grudging semicooperation between the formerly warring entities molecularly replaced obstinate obstructionism, it increased the likelihood of more families receiving concrete data—and mortal remains—therefore enabling them to bury, grieve, and mourn for their dead.

Finally, families of the missing in Bosnia created powerful NGOs, such as the Mothers of Srebrenica and Zepa.[14] They demanded that their governments and the international community focus *equally* on punishing the perpetrators of crimes against humanity *and* identifying all the missing.

The Emergence of Forensic Science in the Finding, Investigation, and Identification of the Dead

Forensic science analyses of the mortal remains of the missing in war are a very recent development. In 1976 a military junta overthrew the Argentinean government and immediately went after left-wing "subversive" groups and individuals who opposed the dictatorship. Students, professors, news reporters, journalists, and lawyers disappeared. Transported to one of 360 detention centers, they were tortured and killed in bestial ways. More than ten thousand persons seized during the seven years died in the detention centers. Many of the bodies found their way into mass graves spread across Argentina.

In 1984, one year after Argentina's "Guerra Sucia" (Dirty War) ended, the new government asked a human rights medical expert with the American Association for the Advancement of Science (AAAS), Eric Stover, to help Argentineans find the thousands who disappeared in that seven-year conflict (1976–1983). Stover accepted and, with the assistance of Dr. Clyde Snow (who is called the "father of Forensic Anthropology"[15]) began to pull together the needed forensic experts. The request followed nearly a year of weekly rallies organized by the NGO, Mothers and Grandmothers of the Plaza de Mayo, and held in Buenos Aires. They demanded that the government find their disappeared family members.

Stover and Snow arrived in Argentina with some forensic anthropologists to train Argentinean medical students and doctors and to create a forensic NGO—the first of its kind, the Argentine Forensic Anthropology Team (EAAF).[16]

There is a two-pronged goal for the EAAF: first, to recover, identify, and assure an appropriate burial for the dead;

and second, to compile evidence of atrocities, war crimes, and crimes against humanity and deliver the data to the office of the state prosecutor for indictment and trial of the perpetrators.

These have been the goals of *all* the NGOs created after 1984. One dozen years later, the PHR, created in 1986, and the EAAF forensic specialists arrived in Bosnia to begin the still-continuing tasks of finding, determining the cause of death, and identifying the mortal remains. At the same time, the newly created ICMP began similar forensic work in Bosnia, in cooperation with other NGOs and Bosnian forensic specialists. The ICRC has worked in a cooperative manner with these forensic NGOs to try to reach some kind of closure for the families of the missing.

These NGOs have, since their creation in the 1980s and 1990s, worked in dozens of war zones across the globe to find and identify the disappeared. And new forensic organizations were established in nations such as Guatemala and Chile, which experienced war and revolution.[17] The newly organized NGOs work closely with already established forensic groups—from their start-up needs to cooperative forensic fieldwork. All new forensic NGOs have been assisted by Eric Stover, Dr. Snow, and their colleagues in the organization and training of the local forensic specialists.

Included in the forensic sciences community are the following major subfields: anthropology, archeology, pathology, biology, botany, genetics, entomology, geology, and odontology. The forensic anthropologist (FA) is probably the most important scientist working in Bosnia many years after the disappearances. The FA is trained in physical anthropology, with a special emphasis on osteology, the study of bones. She scientifically analyzes the skeletal remains that may become evidence in criminal proceedings in the ICTY or in a state criminal court. Studying skeletal remains tells the scientist a great deal about the cause of death. The FA is trained in fields "beyond skeletal biology. Knowledge of medical and legal terminology and procedures is essential [for they] increasingly must communicate with other team members in the course of discovery, in the autopsy suite, and in the courtroom."[18]

They work in gruesome circumstances—the putrid smell of the gravesite inhabits their clothing, their skin, their hair. They use trowels, shovels, picks, and chopsticks, when necessary, to remove the dirt and debris from the bodies they have discovered and are exhuming.

The forensic archeologist is also an important member of the FA community. His primary task in Bosnia is finding the location of the mass graves and scientifically extracting the remains found in them. He works closely with the forensic anthropologists in this important part of the exhumation process. The extraction must be carefully done, especially when the recovery involves secondary mass graves containing disarticulated portions of human remains. Everything must be measured, recorded, and photographed before the remains are placed in a body bag for removal to a morgue.

The forensic pathologist generally is a medical doctor who has studied and interned in medical schools and performs autopsies of dead persons to determine the cause of death. The pathologist's focus, a very limited one in the Bosnian scenario, is on the soft tissue of the victim (which includes analysis of the organs and body fluids of the dead person). Since bones as well as human cadavers are brought into the morgue, the forensic pathologist generally works with a forensic anthropologist.

Forensic entomologists, experts who study arthropods (including flies, beetles, and other insects), help in the death investigation process by determining the intervals between when the death of the victims occurred, when the mass grave was dug, and when the dead were buried. Forensic botanists bring their knowledge of plants into play when they analyze evidence obtained from plants. They are able to determine whether a body has been moved from one gravesite to another as well as using their knowledge to detect hidden mass gravesites. A forensic geologist is also employed in forensic teams because the study of soils can produce evidence linking an individual to a particular place or gravesite. Forensic odontologists use their dentistry experience to assist in the identification of the victim's age and to analyze trauma to the jaw and teeth of the victim.[19]

However, experienced forensic scientists are often pressed into service in other areas of forensic work because of their team's unexpected and urgent need. It is not unusual for a forensic odontologist to serve as the team's pathologist.

Who are the forensic specialists who have been toiling in the killing fields since 1995? The next section examines the lives of seven men and women from the United States, Finland, and Bosnia.

The Stories of Seven Forensic Specialists Working in Bosnia

Based on my conversations with a number of the forensic specialists who worked at the gravesites and in Bosnia's mortuaries, I came to an acute appreciation of their work. What follows are sketches of seven men and women from across the forensic specialists spectrum, whom I have met in person or through their professional writings. While they come from different countries, are of all ages, and have different tasks, they and the hundreds of their colleagues who work in Bosnia share a common goal: to discover and identify *all* the missing and end the suffering of the survivors.

Amor Masovic, Bosniak, MPI Director

Amor Masovic is a citizen of Bosnia, born in Sarajevo in 1955. He went to law school at the University of Sarajevo and practiced law in that city from 1983 to 1992. During the war years (1992–1995), Masovic served as president of the State Commission for the Exchange of Prisoners of War of the government of the Republic of Bosnia and Herzegovina. This meant that he negotiated with the other warring entities for prisoner exchanges. Needless to say, that was a very grueling and frustrating job for Masovic.

In 1995, after the Dayton Peace Accords ended the war,[20] he was appointed chairman of the State Commission for Search for Missing Persons of the newly created (at Dayton) state of Bosnia and Herzegovina (Bosnia).[21] The commission was desperately needed to assist surviving family members locate their missing kinfolk. Staffed by fewer than two dozen men, all Bosniaks, their task was a gruesome one: to assist in locating the mass and individual gravesites, exhume the remains, and then try to identify the skeletons and the cause of death.

In 2000 the commission became the Institute for Missing Persons (IMP), but with no change in its essential task: the identification of the exhumed mortal remains of war victims. In August 2005, at the insistence of the ICMP, the Bosnian Council of Ministers established the Missing Persons Institute (MPI).

Its task was not unchanged; however, its activities encompassed the finding of *all* mass graves hidden by Serbs *and by Croats and Bosniaks* as well as identifying the remains of *all* the dead. This necessitated a new organization encompassing the wartime actions of both entities in the new nation. It meant that the Bosnian Croat-Muslim Federation and the Republika Srpska administrators, politicians, and bureaucrats had to work cooperatively to complete their fundamental task.

The MPI replaced the IMP, although Masovic remained one of the three directors. In 2014 he still remains one of the three directors (the other two are a Bosnian Croat and a Bosnian Serb, the latter appointed by the government of the Republika Srpska). Masovic still often works seven days a week, many times up to eighteen hours a day.

As president of the IMP and director of the MPI, Masovic's administrative work was and remains enormous. It consists of keeping records of the missing, recording and identifying bodily remains, and cooperating with local courts as well as the ICTY prosecutor's office in the multifaceted identification process. Masovic must also work with the UN's specialized agencies such as the UNHCR, the UN Special Envoy for Human Rights, the ICRC Work Group, IFOR and SFOR representatives, a variety of local, national, and international NGOs working in Bosnia, and the forensic teams from the ICMP and the PHR.

Masovic is an important administrator, but he is more than that. He still works in the field with forensic personnel discovering new gravesites and working to bring the bones up from their oftentimes deep tombs. He "leads Bosnia's mass-grave search and has dug burial sites for nearly a decade." He is recognized across Bosnia and, at police checkpoints, "they wave him by. On the street people spontaneously greet him and give thanks."[22]

During the war, he tried to find Bosniak prisoners held by the Serbs. With the war's end, Masovic's task changed somewhat: he was still trying to find Bosniaks, but they were probably dead. Searching for the disappeared had become Masovic's life work. "For as long as there are missing," he said to me in May 2003, "I will continue to look for them." A few years later, he told a reporter: "I only regret that I can't find them all, despite how long we search."[23]

On many occasions, the entire Masovic family, his wife Aida, his daughter Negra, and son Omar travel with him. He has even had Omar work with him at the exhumation sites themselves, where the mortal remains have been found.

Asked why he brought teenage son with him into the caves, pits, and ravines where the bodies were hidden, Masovic's answer was intense: "I wanted to give my child a chance [to see the reality of the war] so that he is prepared. My son knows, he has seen. I told him: 'The circumstances are such that in school you'll have to respond the way it's written in your textbooks; you should say that, but you know, it's in your head, you've seen.' He saw a girl aged three or four in Hrgar. She was pulled out from 66 meters under the surface, and we never identified her.[24] We know that she is a girl, we found her boots. . . . He saw with his own eyes."[25]

He literally goes to newly discovered sites and works with his colleagues and forensic personnel to carefully uncover and remove bones of missing victims from the Bosnian war. Since 1995 Masovic has actively participated in the processes of search and exhumation of more than fifteen thousand mortal remains. They have been exhumed from 290 "mass" (5–300 victims) and more than 3,500 "individual" (1–4 victims) gravesites, including victims tossed into deep natural caves in the Bosnian countryside.

Sanela Bajrambasic, Bosniak: ICRC Spokesperson

Working cooperatively with Masovic and the MPI is the world's first international NGO, the ICRC. Its Balkan Work Group is located in Sarajevo and ten other locations in Bosnia. The ICRC began its labor in 1992 and is still in country, beginning its third decade. The primary tasks of the ICRC in Bosnia are to assist surviving family members to find their missing kin and to support the survivors by providing "psychological-social" counseling and assistance.

Heading the group working with Masovic in 2003 (when I met them) was another former Bosnian lawyer, then-thirty-two-year-old Sanela Bajrambasic, a pretty, somewhat shy, dirty-blond native. She had been working on this task of finding the "disappeared" since 1995. She developed two AMD methods that aided in the undertaking. The first innovation was the NGO's "Book of Missing Persons in the Territory of Bosnia." As she told me, the ICRC "regularly publishes" the names of the missing persons, sorted in alphabetical order and by place and date of disappearance. When we met in her office, five editions of this book had already been published. The first edition, published in 1996, contained eleven thousand names; the fifth edition contained more than seventeen thousand names of people "whose fate was partially clarified [place and date of disappearance were known] but," she said, "their human remains have not been found yet." In 2010 there were still nearly fifteen thousand names listed in the latest edition of the book, which is distributed to the entities in Bosnia as well as to all other NGOs working in the country, such as the ICMP and the PHR.[26]

The second device she established was the "Book of Belongings," a rectangular-shaped book displaying photographs of articles of clothing and artifacts found when the bodies were exhumed from the graves. Sanela and other ICRC and ICMP professionals sit with survivors as the family members pore over the pictures in an effort to find something that their brother, husband, father, or uncle wore or possessed (a watch or a ring) when they disappeared.

Like Amor, Sanela travels a great deal and works long, hard hours. While Masovic, when not functioning as an administrator, works on finding and exhuming the cadavers, Sanela ministers to the surviving family members who very much want to identify their loved ones in order to reach closure on their personal tragedies. Finding, identifying, and, finally, burying their loved ones will, hopefully, allow the survivors to resume a "normal" life. Until they know the fate of their disappeared, they cannot forget.

Moreover, like Masovic, Sanela told me that she will continue to do this work even though the emotional burdens are often great—on her and her colleagues. In her second decade on the job, Sanela is the ICRC spokesperson for its Sarajevo Delegation. She meets with representatives of SFOR, ICMP, MPI, various UN delegations, and local NGOs such as the Mothers of Sarajevo and Zepa.

At the same time, as the delegation's broadcast media representative, she has traveled across Bosnia to write short essays and produce radio reports about the efforts of the ICRC in the state to aid the survivors.[27] Her life is consumed in helping the families of the disappeared find their missing.

Clea Koff, American, Forensic Anthropologist

Clea Koff, born in 1972 in Great Britain, is a mixed-race, Jewish daughter of a Tanzanian mother and an American father. Both parents are documentary filmmakers who focus on authenticating human rights violations; they have traveled around the globe and always have taken Clea and her brother with them. Clea's early school years were spent in England, Kenya, Tanzania, Somalia, and the United States.

She said, at age seven, that she "pictured herself in a highly ordered world. I was always organizing or dreaming of organizing things."[28] She did not know that she would be spending her life organizing different people's bones across the world in the effort to explain what had happened to them. She "grew up to bring order to the contents of mass graves."[29]

When she was a teenager, her father gave Clea a book that changed her life. It was Clyde Snow's *Witnesses from The Grave* and told the story of the creation of the Argentine Forensic Anthropology Team in 1983 and its initial search for the thousands of "disappeared" in that nation. Although when she was younger she yearned to be a librarian, *Witnesses* changed her dramatically. "I basically carried that book around all the time for years. I was insane. I cold-called people at the FBI and would say, 'I'm 18 years old, and I want to study forensics, and I'm looking one day to volunteer for the Argentine team.'"[30]

She came away from her reading of the book with one critical message: bones have stories to tell and "all they need is someone to tell it."[31] She devoted herself to follow the example of her parents—to work on behalf of human rights.

By the time she entered high school in California, she was committed to studying human osteology (the study of the structure and function of the 206 bones in the human body). As she said to an interviewer years later: "I have an innate excitement about bones. They speak to me. [As her mentor, Dr. Clyde Snow, said], 'Bones don't lie,' I like that."[32]

She earned her bachelor's degree in anthropology from Stanford University in 1995 and immediately began work on a master's degree in forensic anthropology at the University of Arizona.

While working over the summer of 1996 at Berkeley, Clea, only twenty-three years old, was invited to become a member of the first ever, sixteen-member forensic team—consisting of forensic anthropologists, archeologists, and pathologists—to collect evidence of war crimes and crimes against humanity for the Prosecutor's Office of the International Criminal Tribunal for Rwanda (ICTR) and the ICTY.

In order to indict and prosecute those responsible for these crimes in these war zones, the prosecutors needed proof that the bodies found in graves were noncombatants who were murdered. And so, in 1995, the ICTR/Y prosecutor, Richard Goldstone, asked the PHR to form the team to investigate the mass graves in Africa and the Balkans.

She immediately accepted the invitation and, over the next five years, served on seven forensic teams that worked in Rwanda (two) and in the former Yugoslavia (five). During the time between forensic assignments, Clea finished her master's work in forensic anthropology in 1999 and received her degree from the University of Nebraska.

The missions to Croatia, Bosnia, and Kosovo, conducted between 1996 and 2001, brought Koff into close contact with the terrible stench of the reality of war, war crimes, and crimes against humanity. As she wrote in her book, *The Bone Woman*, after unearthing the remains of murdered Bosniak civilians—hands tied behind their backs—she "felt anger toward people who deem murder an acceptable political policy. I felt the last of my naïveté drain away as I uncovered more and more people shot while their hands were tied. And I felt two kinds of duty—to identify them and allow them to incriminate their killers; and the other to their relatives—to help return the remains to them."[33]

As with all the forensic specialists working in these post-war killing fields, Koff suffered from the work she was doing for the prosecutor's office. Most of the time, however, she steeled herself while working in the field or in the morgue.

But there were times when she broke down while working with the bodies. For example, she recalled how she felt after successfully identifying the body of a young boy. Protocol prevented Clea from telling the parents. "I felt bad for him and for everyone in the world. The loss of my 'professional distance' shocked me.'"[34]

Particular words written down ("bullet, left maxilla" and "homicide") many times daily often led to the emotional outpouring of tears by the forensic workers. Glances by survivors observing the excavation of a mass gravesite triggered tears. "To see funerals made me cry," Clea wrote.[35]

There were also those times when the professionals broke down in front of their colleagues, and it affected all of them. Koff recalled a Swedish forensic anthropologist in great pain after working on the body of a young child. The woman left her work station and ran out crying. Clea joined her outside. "Waving her hand back towards the morgue, she said: 'I have never seen anything like that before. It's just a child . . . how? . . . why?' Why was she there if she was going to force me to contemplate—during the working day—the bleak and harsh reality of the dead, when I had to go back inside and keep up my end of things for another month? I was thinking, 'Don't do this to me. Don't start me crying, because I might never stop.'"[36]

Eventually, the grisly environment forced Koff to end her work in Bosnia. In 2005 she founded the Missing Persons Identification Resource Center, an NGO based in Los Angeles, California. Its task is to link families in the United States who have missing persons with the coroner's office in LA. (The morgue holds a great number of unidentified bodies.) She still works with bones but far from mass gravesites in the Balkans.

Irfanka Pasagic, Bosniak, Psychotherapist, President/founder, Tuzlanska Amica (NGO)

Wars always lead to traumatization of participants and innocents alike. In the Bosnian wars, the civilian population experienced massive, sustained brutality and human rights violations throughout the four years of war. "Civilians were both the instrument and the target of war, [enduring] numerous highly traumatic situations and gross abuses."[37] This "human induced trauma, e.g., war or abuse, leaves especially deep mental scars. If the injury is inflicted by a familiar person and is not anticipated, the traumatisation is especially prolonged as a result. If it is accompanied by sexual assault, the impacts are always devastating, affecting many survivors for the rest of their lives."[38] In the Bosnian wars, both factors were present: neighbors killed neighbors, and thousands of Bosniak women were brutally raped by the enemy.

Dr. Irfanka Pasagic has worked as a clinical psychologist and has researched and written scholarly reports about the psychological consequences of the Bosnian war. Born in Srebrenica, Bosnia, in 1953, Irfanka went to medical school in Zagreb, Croatia, specializing in neurology and psychiatry. She did postgraduate studies in psychotherapy at Gothenburg University, Sweden, and studied trauma education at the University of Missouri.

She began practicing medicine in 1979 in her hometown, where she headed the Center for Rehabilitation and Hematology from 1986 to 1992. When the Bosnian war began in 1992, she and thousands of other Bosniaks were deported from Srebrenica to the Bosniak-held city of Tuzla, located in the northeastern part of Bosnia. The city quickly added many more refugees over the next three years.

By 1995, there were 150,000 people trying to survive in Tuzla: 60 percent were refugees from areas captured by the Bosnian Serb armies. The great majority of the new arrivals—mostly women and children, widows and war orphans—lived in terrible conditions and suffered from the trauma brought on by the war.

As soon as Dr. Pasagic arrived in Tuzla, she knew that the new arrivals needed material help to survive. She also knew that, more importantly, these survivors needed medical assistance, especially psychological support, to deal with the consequences of the traumas they experienced at the hands of the Bosnian Serbs.

The major problem for the survivors, Pasagic writes, is the destruction of the family, both the immediate one and the communal one—the village. Psychotherapists working with the survivors "say that their patients continue to see themselves only as part of something bigger—the wife in a family, or a member of a village—never as an individual. Pasagic, a psychiatrist who has worked with these women, said, 'From the time she could speak, the woman was told in words and examples that her value was based on what a man thought of her.'"[39]

In 2006 Dr. Pasagic said, "The society in which the survivors lived no longer exists as such. In its stead, a form of collective traumatization emerges. . . . The family structure under such circumstances is very disturbed and has

FORENSIC SCIENTISTS AT WORK

very significant negative consequences, in particular for children. [Since most missing and dead are the male family members], the role of the woman in the family is the one that changes especially and she, with her own trauma, must assume new responsibilities. Often she is the only source of support for the surviving family members."[40]

The consequences for women of their changed position in society are difficult and traumatic ones. Most of these women have never gone to school beyond the fourth grade, never left their village, or held a job prior to the war. "We were responsible for the house, the men had everything outside," said one widow after the war.[41]

Thousands of them were victims of rape during the war and "many never leave their houses because of the shame they feel." Furthermore, because there are still so many war criminals free in Bosnia, "there are many places . . . where victim and criminal live next to each other. Many children," Pasagic writes, "are growing up knowing that persons who killed their fathers or brothers live normal lives."[42] However, these Bosniak women must somehow overcome their traumas and keep the remaining family members together in the face of the ugly reality of postwar life in Bosnia.

For them and for their children, school is one major key to survival. Dr. Pasagic notes, sadly, that many of the teachers trying to help the surviving children "are traumatized by the war themselves. During training sessions, some teachers end up in tears, she said. 'It is very difficult to expect someone with trauma to work on people with trauma. You can't go through four years of war without trauma. There's nobody among them who hasn't lost somebody. Before they can help children, someone has to help [the teachers].'"[43]

For Dr. Pasagic, perhaps the only way to reach these traumatized children is through the schools. "For many children who survived Srebrenica, when they arrived in Tuzla [in July 1995], their first question was, 'When does school start?' Irfanka said. "It's the only part of their life that's the same as before the war. They have no home, they've lost their families—the only place they feel some kind of normalcy is school."[44]

From the "very beginning of her experiences as a refugee and as psychiatrist, Irfanka has proved remarkably sensitive and sensible in finding ways of helping displaced people. . . . She struggled so that children could be included in women assistance projects, and repeatedly pointed out the lack of projects specifically aimed at giving psychological help to men."[45]

In 1992 she formed the Group for Psychological Assistance to Traumatized Women and Camp Detainees. This NGO provided one-on-one psychological assistance to these women and to their children. In 1994 Dr. Pasagic began her work as supervisor of a UNICEF project, "Woman and Child," supported by a Norwegian NGO, Norwegian People's Aid. She supervised twenty other psychotherapists as they went about the task of addressing the problems of these patients. In 1996 she assisted in the creation and operation of Tuzlanska Amica, the NGO that supports and aids women and children traumatized in the war in Bosnia. In 1999 Irfanka became president of the NGO.

The group's work, led by psychotherapists under the supervision of Dr. Pasagic, includes education and supervision for a number of long-term projects focused on the mental and physical health of the women and children. In 2015 these projects included:

1. Summer volunteer camps for children, where the young survivors enjoy creative activities while also receiving help from professionals for their trauma. These organized activities take place in refugee camps and the Tuzla orphanage.

2. An outpatient department for children, which is a free service offered by doctors who provide checkups of orphans and children who are not in primary school. More than one thousand such medical treatments take place monthly in Tuzla's Health House.

3. Distance Adoption, in which more than one thousand children have thus far been "adopted," mainly by Italian families, at a cost of thirty euros a month.

4. Nutritional Aid Program, which addresses the immense nutritional deficiencies in the diets of children of the many poor refugees living in Tuzla.

5. Mobile Teams who visit the recipients of assistance from overseas families to give them the funds they badly need to survive.

6. The Tuzla Orphanage, established and run by the government. The long-distance "adoption" program established by the NGO supports it. Currently, there are more than two hundred Bosnian children living in the facility.

7. When children living in the Orphanage reach age eighteen, they must leave the house. However, there is a facility, Family House, for a small number of eighteen-year-olds Bosnian youths.

8. Medical care in Italy for women and children who cannot be successfully treated in Bosnia.

9. The House of Friendship, another establishment created by Tuzlanska Amica, located in Brcko, with recreational and educational activities for children and youths of all ages.[46]

In addition to her psychological assistance to these women and children, Dr. Pasagic has engaged in research, writing, and participation in conferences around the globe that focus on the problems faced by innocent civilians—

women, children, and men—in Bosnia, Rwanda, and other war zones. Her article, one of two dozen she has authored, on the traumatic experiences among women in Bosnia during the war is a standard reference for scholars and practitioners.[47]

Since 1993 she has been an active leader in the *Project Bridges between Women*. In 1995 she founded *Human Rights Office Tuzla*. Her efforts have brought together psychotherapists from Sweden, Norway, Germany, Italy, and the United States to address these grim medical/social/psychological issues. In 1998, along with another psychotherapist, Dr. Yael Danieli, she initiated another NGO: *Democracy Cannot Be Built with the Hands of Broken Souls*. The major goals of the project "were to establish a dialogue between the different groups [Bosniaks and Bosnian Serbs] at different levels and to prevent the conspiracy of silence."[48]

Dr. Pasagic cares passionately about her patients. In 2007, for example, she canceled her appearance at a conference at The Hague. The panel's chairperson announced that Dr. Pasagic was not able to come at the last minute "as a result of the anguish of the many victims she counsels following on from the decision of the International Court of Justice [*Bosnia v Serbia and Montenegro*[49]]." Her statement noted: "Survivors, rushing these days into my office having lost even the ultimate hope that the world will confess the horrible crime committed upon them and clearly name the responsible ones, have definitely made me decide not to come to The Hague. I think it is here where I am needed more."[50]

Dr. Pasagic continues her work with traumatized patients in Bosnia and other nations facing these problems. She keeps on contributing to the profession's understanding of trauma brought on by war through her research and her work with other humanitarian organizations across the world. For her ongoing humanitarian work since 1992, Dr. Pasagic received the International Award of the Alexander

Langer Foundation in 2005 for her work as a bridge-building peace activist.

Eric Stover, American, Forensic Science Team Administrator,
U N "Expert on Mission," Bosnia

Eric Stover, presently the director of the Human Rights Center at the University of California, Berkeley, is also Adjunct Professor of Law and Public Health and member of the Joint Medical Program there.

Being born in 1954 in Detroit, Michigan, and then living in small farm towns in the Midwest does not account for his commitment to working for human rights worldwide. In a revealing interview in 1999, Stover admitted his "fascination with the darker side of life and what happened to people." He remembers, when he was six or seven years old, watching a newsreel on the Holocaust and asking, "How could this sort of barbarity happen?"[51]

He admits that the French existentialist Albert Camus greatly influenced his life. Stover calls himself an "'absurdist,' aligning his world view with Camus' theory of absurdism [i.e.], that things are going to happen and there are a lot of things you can't control, but if you learn to focus yourself and if you have strong principles and interests, then you can accomplish something."[52]

After what he claims was a "misspent youth" traveling across Europe and working as a journalist, he "learned to focus" himself and began to act on the "dark" issue he saw when he was young: how and why did barbarity happen and what could a person do to mitigate that evil. His first human rights work was a job with Amnesty International in London. That experience sent Stover on the focused path he has followed since then.

Since the 1970s he has written books and essays about human rights abuses and has been associated with a number of major human rights N G Os including Amnesty International (AI), Human Rights Watch (HRW), Physicians for Human Rights (PHR), and the Human Rights program of the American Association for the Advancement of Science (AAAS).

His research interests, reflected in his writings and his activism, are the medical and social consequences of war; forensic sciences and war crimes investigations; justice and reconstruction in the aftermath of mass violence; and infectious diseases and human rights. Stover is also on the advisory boards of a number of human rights associations, including the Journal of Health and Human Rights, Harvard School of Public Health; the Robert F. Kennedy Human Rights Award; Humanity United, Omidyar Foundation[53]; and the John D. and Catherine T. MacArthur Foundation's Trust Fund for War-Affected Children in Northern Uganda.

Stover organized the first forensic teams that journeyed to Bosnia in 1993. He labels those first forays into the Balkan wars "flak jacket" forensic anthropology. As he said: "It was grim work and, at times, dangerous. One shot from a sniper's rifle or an RPG (rocket propelled grenade) lobbed down from the hills could bring the whole operation to a screeching halt."[54] There were times when "the grisly task [exhuming the bodies] was interrupted by a rain of rocket shells. 'That,' Stover acidly notes, '*focuses* your attention.'"[55]

For Stover and other members of the forensic teams, "such extraordinary occupational hazards—among other misfortunes, he's been stricken with hepatitis in Bosnia and arrested by both the Argentine and Serbian militaries, the latter hauling him off to jail as UN peacekeepers watched—come with the territory."[56] Stover, however, is embarrassed when people say forensic work in these war-ravaged areas requires courage. His mocking response: "my wife might say [it requires] stupidity."[57]

At the time, the early 1990s, Stover was the executive director of another major NGO, PHR. Since the ICTY's creation in 1993, he has served on a number of medicolegal forensic investigations as a UN-designated "Expert on Mission."

The requests, coming from the ICTY prosecutor's office, were to investigate and discover the evidence needed to issue indictments against those responsible for the numerous mass killings of Bosniaks and Croats. The essential problem for those prosecuting perpetrators of war crimes and crimes against humanity in Bosnia was different from the one facing prosecutors at the Nuremberg War Crimes Tribunal in 1945. At Nuremberg, the prosecutors had massive amounts of data incriminating the Nazi perpetrators. In Bosnia there were few documents illuminating the brutal policy the perpetrators followed. "Because the Balkan offenders," Stover wrote, "did not keep meticulous records of their bloody deeds, prosecutors have needed a substantial number of eyewitnesses to make their charges stick."[58]

There were eyewitnesses to the brutality. However, what the ICTY prosecutor's office greatly needed from the forensic scientists were, first, finding and identifying victims *in order to corroborate eyewitness testimony*, and second, *determining how the victim died.*[59]

As executive director of the PHR, Stover recruited and shuttled nearly one hundred scientists into and out of the former Yugoslavia to work in these killing fields. It quickly "developed into the largest international forensic investigation of war crimes—or possibly of any crime—in history."[60]

This was not the first time Stover organized forensic teams to look into the disappearance of victims of war's cruelty and killing. His initial involvement with forensic work in this area was in Argentina. During that country's "dirty war" waged by the military dictatorship against socialists, communists, and their supporters, many thousands of citizens—between nine thousand and thirty thousand—disappeared. After the junta fell in 1983, there quickly developed the need for some kind of medical organization to help Argentineans find the missing.

At that very moment, Stover headed the human rights program of the American Association for the Advancement of Science (AAAS). Representatives of an Argentinean NGO visited Stover in Washington DC to ask him to help them find and identify their missing family members. They came because bodies were being exhumed from mass graves, but there was no scientific process that could identify them. "And so," Stover recalled, "I was asked by both the NGO and by the Alfonsin government, to come in and to train a team to carry out the exhumation in a proper fashion."[61]

However, there was a problem. Stover knew next to nothing about forensics. After consulting with the National Academy of Forensic Sciences, he met with Clyde Snow, the leading forensic anthropologist in America. With Snow's help, as well as the assistance of a world-famous geneticist, Mary Claire King, a multidisciplinary team went to Argentina to train an Argentinean team of medical students. The team Stover and Snow put together consisted of a forensic radiologist, archeologist, anthropologist, odontologist, and a pathologist. The idea was a simple one: "Take scientific knowledge that had evolved out of the departments of anthropology and criminology and apply them in this area where human rights violations are occurring."[62] He worked in the field in 1983 and 1984. In June 1984, Stover testified for the prosecution at the trial of leaders of the military junta.[63]

Argentina became the first nation to use forensic scientists to find and identify the missing, and provide incriminating evidence to state prosecutors for possible criminal action. After 1983 forensic scientists found themselves working in other nations beset by war and revolution, including Guatemala, Iraq, Rwanda, and, beginning in 1995, Bosnia.

Srebrenica's tragic events greatly affected Stover. There,

uncovering the remains of thousands of victims of Bosnian Serb war crimes, he "fully realized" the devastation "felt by people who are unable to identify their lost or 'disappeared' family members."[64]

"That was a deep learning moment for me. The ICTY was supposed to be working for these victims. But the thing family members want most is identification of these bodies. More than justice, they want proper burial."[65] And this reality underscored, for Stover and the forensic scientists, the symbiotic relationship that developed between them and the families of the disappeared. The forensic teams, he said, "become very much involved with the families and witnesses and who this person is whom you are trying to identify, and you also become involved with the families."[66] Whenever they can, family members visit the gravesites and watch the forensic scientists work to uncover and exhume the bodies.

"Eventually," Stover notes, "the team members begin interacting with the families. They'll talk to a family member. Sometimes the families will bring photographs of their missing relatives. [This interaction] has a profound effect on how they view the world. You see a change in the forensic scientists themselves, which is important."[67]

Stover and others experience horrible nightmares. Their work takes an emotional toll.[68] Nevertheless, there are rewards as well and, for many forensic scientists, the benefits far outweigh the negatives of forensic work.

> When I'm asked about the "grisly work of exhumations" and so on—and I mean this sincerely—it's a privilege. Because even though in Argentina or Guatemala or Bosnia you enter through a dark portal into those societies and cultures, it is a real need. Families want the remains returned. . . . And what they need is a tool. You're bringing them that tool. And you're learning from them. It's like non-biological family in many

countries, because I've gotten to know these families so well. So it's a privilege in the sense that you're engaged with people in a way that most people in their jobs don't get to be.[69]

Why dig up the mass graves? So history is set straight, answered Stover. Physical evidence of war crimes uncovered by the forensic scientists puts the lies of the perpetrators to rest. The evidence, placed alongside witness testimony, is the basis for convicting the perpetrators in the criminal courts. Finally, he said, from a "humanitarian perspective, the digging process provides families of the missing [with knowledge] of the fate of their loved ones and [enables them] to give them a proper burial."[70]

Eric Stover's focus remains sharp and unambiguous, as his decades of forensic human rights work attest. Over a lifetime, Stover knows the "importance of being actively involved on the ground, applying science-slash-technology in the service of human rights."[71]

Helena Banta, Finn, Forensic Odontologist

Helena Ranta is a dentist who, in 1993, at the age of 48, serendipitously became a forensic odontologist. Traveling home from Norway, she stopped to visit a friend in Stockholm, Sweden. While she was there a tragedy occurred: a car ferry sank in the Gulf of Finland, killing hundreds of passengers. Many of the dead were police officers and forensic workers. Because she spoke Swedish, Banta was asked to stay and help identify the victims. With that forensic work, Ranta's life changed forever. In an understated reflection on her life, she said, "When I was younger I imagined my life to be very different. I thought it would be easier."[72]

That year, Elisabeth Rehn, a UN Human Rights rapporteur, found out about the discovery of dozens of unburied bodies on a hillside in Kravica, Bosnia. Contacted by Rehn, Dr. Ranta and a forensic team she pulled together traveled to the Balkans to investigate the deaths. Since then, Helena's forensic team—consisting only of Finnish experts—has exhumed and identified the remains and provided physical evidence to prosecutors across the globe. Bosnia, Kosovo, Peru, Colombia, Cameroon, Nepal, Iraq, and Chechnya are some of the war zones she has worked in since 1993.

She believes that UN prosecutors and other governmental agencies who need help finding, exhuming, and identifying the cause of death of the disappeared ask for her assistance because of her and her nation's reputation. "We Finns have been tolerated even in places where representatives of great powers have been unwelcome. Perhaps we are easy to accept. . . . Finland has no colonial past and is not a member of NATO. We have convinced the international community. [They] believe that we are unbiased and that we cannot be influenced. There is no point trying to bribe me. Or threaten me. Or blackmail me."[73]

Ranta, like other forensic scientists, "dodged snipers' bullets, negotiated with military commanders who looked like highway robbers, dug for decomposing corpses in graves, and built entire skeletons out of bone fragments. She once ordered U.S. forces to use their tanks to protect her working group."[74] Before and after exhumation work, especially in Bosnia and Kosovo, Ranta received death threats. However, she is a strong woman, undeterred by them. "I sleep well at night. If there are threats, there are arrangements for dealing with them."[75]

Ranta has done things in her work as a forensic team leader that were unimaginable prior to 1993. "She has smuggled dead bodies in the former Yugoslavia[76] and been a witness in the trial of Slobodan Milosevic at the UN's ICTY at The Hague."[77]

Testifying in 2003 in The Hague in the Milosevic trial, Ranta used the data she and her Finnish forensic team collected in 1999 and 2000. Ironically, Milosevic himself had invited the Finnish forensic experts into Serbia in January 1999 to investigate the deaths of more than forty ethnic Albanians in Racak, Kosovo (then a province of Serbia). Ranta recalled, "The international community had really started to pressure Milosevic and he did not have many alternatives. [He had to make a choice] between two bad alternatives, [and he chose] the less dangerous [forensic group]. And what would seem less dangerous than a small team of researchers from the Department of Forensic Medicine at the University of Helsinki, especially as the team is led by a woman."[78]

The Racak event was a "turning point" in the Kosovo war. It unfolded in dramatic fashion. On January 16, 1999, the head of the Organization of Security and Cooperation in Europe (OSCE), William Walker, on a cease-fire verification mission to Kosovo, found twenty-three bodies in a ditch outside the village of Racak. All told, forty-five bodies were taken to Pristina, Kosovo, two days later, where autopsies were performed by Serb, Finnish, and Belarusian pathologists.

Dr. Ranta and her team, selected by Milosevic, were part of the group doing the autopsies. She was appointed chief investigator. The Finnish team continued to collect evidence at the killing site as part of their investigation of the incident. However, other events occurred that cut short their fieldwork. They returned to Helsinki in March 1999.

Calling it a massacre of ethnic Albanians by Serb military forces, Walker passed the preliminary autopsy reports to the EU in March 1999. However, the Finnish forensic experts had not yet reached that conclusion and did not allocate any blame in their preliminary findings. The interim report noted that there was no fighting in Racak and "that the dead civilians had not been carrying weapons."[79]

One week later, NATO unleashed a bombing attack against Serbia. The Ranta report, though incomplete and without any definitive conclusions as to culpability, nevertheless "paved the way for the NATO bombings of Serbia and Kosovo in 1999."[80] By June 1999 Kosovo Implementation Force (KFOR) troops, from NATO countries, were on the ground patrolling the province.

Both sides in the civil war argued their version of the truth vigorously. Kosovars maintained that the dead were unarmed civilians—including women and children—killed by Serb soldiers. The Serbian government insisted that the dead were KLA soldiers killed in battle and that Kosovar Albanians dressed the dead bodies in civilian clothes and claimed that a massacre occurred in Racak. Dr. Ranta's forensic team was "caught squarely in the middle." As she said in 2001: "The work we did was the best possible under those circumstances."

In November 1999 Dr. Ranta's forensic team returned to Racak to continue its investigation into the mass killings. They returned once more in March 2000 to uncover the final pieces of physical evidence (shell-casings, bullets, parts of human remains) for transport to their laboratory in Finland.

The report concluded that twenty-two bodies were discovered in the 3.5–5 meter-wide trench (with one other "nearby"), spread along a distance of 60 meters. Among the dead were a woman and a young child. The killers were behind thick shrub and bushes surrounding the trench. Spent AK-47 shells were picked up from that area. Ballistic analysis indicated that "the victims were shot at a range of less than 30 meters from the trench and then dumped in it."

In the summer of 2000, she submitted the final report, more than one thousand pages long, to the Prosecutor's Office of the ICTY at The Hague. It became the major prosecution weapon in the ICTY's case that Milosevic was responsible for the Racak deaths.

Philosophically, as a medical doctor, Helena Ranta refuses

to use any legal-political or pejorative phrase in her foren-sic reports. One does not see terms such as "massacre," "war crimes," or "genocide" in them. If the physical evi-dence uncovered by her team points to murder, she calls that conclusion a crime against humanity.

A spokesperson for the ICTY's Prosecutor's office explained Ranta's position: "Many expected Ranta to say that it was a massacre. However, she was not a lawyer. Instead, she worked to determine causes of death. Her task as a pathologist was not to define the events in legal terms."[81]

Slobodan Milosevic's trial in The Hague began in Feb-ruary 2002. He faced charges regarding his alleged actions in the former Yugoslavia. Ranta's confrontation with defen-dant Milosevic lasted a number of days and reflected his belief that she bowed to pressure from Western leaders and NATO. Claiming she was "manipulated," he attempted to disprove Ranta's findings that "crimes against humanity" were committed by the Serbs. Milosevic's assertion: the dead were soldiers in the Kosovo Liberation Army killed during battles with the Serbs. They were not civilians mas-sacred by the Serb military. Nearly all the dead had pow-der burn marks on their hands, indicating that they were fighters, not innocent civilians. There were military arti-facts (military identification tag, ammunition container) found by the bodies. Ranta herself, Milosevic argued, "con-spired" with Germany, NATO, and OSCE officials to reach her conclusions.

Ranta countered every one of Milosevic's charges against her personally and against the forensic conclusions reached by the team. She told Milosevic during her tense confron-tation with him in the ICTY that her work in Kosovo "was exclusively to determine the causes of death of those who were killed, without consideration of the possible political repercussions of her report."[82]

Why has she continued to travel mine-laden roads rather

than choose the safe path of practicing dentistry and living safely in a lovely home, surrounded by family and friends? She has a ready answer: "The twentieth century was the century of the culture of impunity. The dead have rights too. I do not look for the guilty parties, but I am one of the many who produce evidence for use in international courts. It is up to them to decide whether the cases in question are genocide, mass murder, or something else."[83]

Dr. Ranta turns down invitations to bring her forensic experts into any country that has capital punishment. "Iraq has reintroduced the death sentence, and that is something I cannot accept under any circumstances. Furthermore, I cannot accept that investigations by forensic scientists I trained might lead to a death sentence."[84]

Since her forays in forensic work began in 1993, Dr. Ranta has become a strong advocate for human rights. (She is a board member of the Finnish League for Human Rights.) This has enabled her to find the strength to continue her forensic work, always confronting mass graves and the gross atrocities she uncovers. She has told many that "[my] concern for human rights is always there in all my work and that lends it meaning. It also helps when you see that your work can—at best—lead to the conviction of the guilty parties so that societies can heal."[85]

At sixty-seven years old, she feels the physical strain more keenly. Ranta remains a professor and team leader of the Finnish Forensic Expert Team. She continues to go into the killing fields but confesses: "I would rather teach [a younger generation of forensic experts] than dig."

Courtney Angela Brkic, Croat-American
Forensic Archeologist; Author

Courtney Brkic is a first-generation American of Croatian descent. Her father is from Croatia, her mother came from Germany, through England. Her father was a youth living in Sarajevo during World War II and told Courtney of his experiences living under Nazi and Ustashe occupation. She brought those memories with her years later when she worked in Croatia and Bosnia.

Born in 1972, she grew up in Arlington, Virginia, and graduated from the College of William and Mary with a degree in archeology. After graduation, she worked as a field archeologist in the eastern United States. In 1995 she received a Fulbright to do research in Croatia, focusing on the effects of the Bosnian war on Croatian women.

Her year in Croatia was a watershed experience for Courtney. One message she received again and again from the many women she met has stayed with her and appears in all her writings about the Bosnian wars: *Their missing will return.*

> Until they are shown evidence, it is a rare person who without evidence can say, I really have to face the fact that most likely [they are dead]. Eventually they have to accept that fact. But it happens because so much time has gone by that it just would defy logic that the person would still be alive. . . . For these women, this situation [not knowing] is shitty. It would be slightly less shitty if I could know. But they did not fool themselves to think that it would be good.[86]

This feeling is the common denominator in these populations, whether the surviving women resided in Guatemala, Argentina, Croatia, or Bosnia. She believes, based on her research and her forensic experiences, that the women "wait first one year, then another. They grow old in their waiting. They reject . . . the conventional wisdom that all is lost."[87]

The Fulbright experience led Brkic to switch her archeological specialization from research and writing to forensic work. In the summer of 1996, when she was twenty-three years old, she decided to return to Bosnia. As she said later,

"I was not seeking experience or adventure. Part of me did not even know why I had come."[88]

She became the forensic archeologist in a team of PHR forensic scientists assigned to exhume and identify the mortal remains of victims in the mass graves at Srebrenica. It was "even more harrowing work" than her year in Croatia, even though it was for a brief two-month period.[89] She was a valuable member of the team because Courtney spoke the language. Because of her inexperience, however, Courtney was a utility player at the Srebrenica sites.

I worked with a forensic team that excavated Srebrenica's mass graves, assisted the forensic pathologists in the morgue in Kalesija with the examinations of the remains, acted as an interpreter for local men we hired to wash clothing from the bodies, and arranged personal effects for a Dutch police photographer. I translated scraps of paper from pockets— prayers, a rare driver's license, the backs of photographs. We found the strangest things: a "Dear John" letter, a bag of salt, a hypodermic needle and ampoules sewn in the lining of a denim jacket. Insulin? We wondered when we found them. Morphine? The men's hands had all been bound with identical lengths of wire.[90]

The exhumation work at the mass graves was difficult, Brkic writes. "The bodies were so enmeshed that it was hard to see which extremity belonged to which corpse. The faces and hands were by far the most difficult, perhaps because clothing covered everything else."[91] She was also very uncomfortable because the forensic staff "felt constantly at the mercy of others—the SFOR soldiers who escorted us to the site, the mines that might or might not be underfoot at any given moment. . . . And I was disturbed by the fact that they were still using the Serb laborers on the grave, probably the same ones who killed the Bosnians [a year ago]."[92]

Like other forensic teams working in Bosnia and Croatia, they had two tasks after finding the locations of the graves: to identify the dead and present the evidence to surviving family members, and to help gather evidence for the ICTY at The Hague. Courtney, because of her work in Croatia a year earlier, "was conscious of the people who were waiting for their missing."[93]

Her labors as a forensic archeologist turned out to be a short-lived career change. As she said years later, "It (forensic archeology) is a morbid and awful pursuit. When I was going out there I thought, 'Maybe I will end up so interested by this that I will go and study this.' *The first day I knew that I was just not cut out for it.*"[94] (my emphasis)

In a 2004 BBC interview, she explained why she left this work: "I had this very personal connection [language and family links], and I think that's ultimately why I decided . . . to leave that work." Although she tried to remain "detached" from her forensic job, the links and her inexperience "meant she became 'immersed' in the past lives of her victims."[95]

Brkic remained involved with the ongoing Bosnian tragedy after she left the killing fields in August 1996. She spent some time working as a translator for the ICTY at The Hague. However, she returned to America, entered New York University's (NYU) Master's in Fine Arts program, and received her MFA degree in 2001.

Since then she has taught creative writing at NYU, Cooper Union, Kenyon College, and George Mason University. She has authored two books focusing on her experiences in the Balkans, *Stillness,*[96] a collection of short stories, and *The Stone Fields*, a memoir of her family's experiences during World War II and of her experiences in 1990s Yugoslavia.

The Physical and Emotional Toll on the Forensic Professionals

Courtney Brkic best reflects the feelings of all the forensic professionals who worked in Bosnia: "At every point,

I didn't see bodies—I saw people. I didn't see articles of clothing; I saw clothing that had been knitted and sewn for these men by women who were waiting for them."[97]

Undoubtedly, working in the killing fields—whether in Bosnia, Rwanda, Somalia, or Guatemala—takes a toll on *all* forensic workers. The physical labor at exhumation sites is strenuous. Twelve-hour days are common and this does not take into account the many hours traveling to and from the work site. Bill Haglund recalled "the overwhelming, exhausting [work], day after day in 1996, eight months straight in graves, between Rwanda and Yugoslavia. I had never been more physically and mentally exhausted [in] my whole life. . . . I felt a tremendous amount of pride just surviving 1996."[98] Dr. Helena Ranta's candid observation is appropriate: forensic work is for the young.

The psychological blows faced by these scientists are more impactful than the physical dangers. David Strinovic, a forensic pathologist working on the human remains of Croatian victims at Vukovar, said what most forensic people probably think:

I'm sure someday I'm going to have psychological problems because of this work. The most painful part is dealing with the mothers. Sometimes they will tell stories about their sons and I become so touched, I start to cry. I can't just remain calm and say to myself, "Okay, be professional, this is just another case which has been solved, now it's time to move on."[99]

Clea Koff, the young forensic anthropologist, began tormenting herself in her dreams and had nightmares because of all the tragedy she was witnessing. Most of the time, these breakdowns occurred after the forensic personnel departed from the killing fields.

As she wrote, the brutally hard work at the site "saves you from thinking and feeling until later, maybe much later, after you have left the mission and you find yourself crying into your pillow 12,000 kilometers away, a world away, with your hands that touched and your mind that remembers that elderly husband and wife [who] are still dead."[100]

Koff said something most forensic personnel would, eventually, certainly agree with. "I felt like I was having trouble looking at bodies as cases. I was having trouble looking at the grave, at the people who lived in the town where I was working. I was feeling bad for everyone all the time. That was making my work very hard to do."[101]

Bill Haglund is a more senior forensic anthropologist. His response to similar horror scenes differed somewhat from Koff's experience. He recalled seeing a mass grave in Rwanda and realized, "You find that there are niches of sensitivity and people react in different ways. [There] was a grave in which about 25 percent, or about 140 of the individuals were children under ten years of age—many babies still wrapped on their mother's back. It's powerful, when you think about it, and your life. I don't think I'm callous, but I realize that if you don't maintain a distance, you can't do your job. I'm armored in some ways by my duties. They armor me."[102]

A broken ankle forced Koff to leave the country in 2001. Although she has testified at criminal trials before the ICTY after her departure from the field, she has not returned to Bosnia. Many forensic workers do not return to the killing fields.

FIVE

The Stark Realities Confronting the Searchers and the Survivors in Bosnia

They say we must all live together now, but I don't know how I can deal with that. I wish my heart would break into pieces. I wish I could die.

—RAMIZA HODZIC

In every one of them [Serbs] I see a murderer.

—JASNA PLOSKIC

In Vukovar you have to wander the streets with a lantern searching for a gentle soul—for people not hardened by hatred and grief.

—BARBARA MATEJCIC

Viewing the events occurring in Bosnia since the end of the war, one sees disturbing events that cast a harsh shadow over the new nation's future. For a great majority of Balkan scholars, the proximate roots of the disarray lay in the arrangement foisted on the warring belligerents—Serbians, Croatians, and Bosniaks—during the intense debates held at an Air Force base from November 1 to 21, 1995.

With the American emissaries, Ambassador Richard Holbrooke and Secretary of State Warren Christopher, leading the discussions and playing hardball with the reluctant Balkan leaders, the 1995 Dayton, Ohio, Peace Accords materialized over twenty-one days in November.

(U.S. Ambassador John C. Kornblum was one of the major drafters of the Accords.[1]) It was formally signed in Paris on December 14, 1995, by the presidents of the major adversaries: Slobodan Milosevic, for the Federal Republic of Yugoslavia *and* the Republika Srpska[2]; Franjo Tudjman, for the Republic of Croatia; Alija Izetbegovic, for Bosnia-Herzegovina; and Fresimir Zubak, for the entity, the Federation of Bosnia-Herzegovina.

From that moment to the present, the peace agreement has been seen as a tool "devised *in extremis* as a war-ending vehicle."[3] The brutal fighting ended with the signing of the Accords. However, the absence of fighting must not be mistaken for stability. While the agreement ended the bloody war, "it was also roundly criticized for rewarding the aggressor and *cementing ethnic tensions into the architecture of the new state*."[4] (my emphasis)

Twenty years after Dayton, in Bosnia, there remains "the absence of a civic conception of state, the ethnicisation of society continues apace, leading many to describe today's divisions as being as wide as at any point since 1995."[5]

In January 2014 James R. Clapper, the director of America's National Intelligence (DNI),[6] told the U.S. Senate Intelligence Committee that Bosnia was one of two explosive European nations: "The situation in Bosnia-Herzegovina and ethnic cleavages in Macedonia are particularly volatile." Repeating the dismal view of that nation's future he had reported one year earlier, Clapper told the senators: In Bosnia-Herzegovina, different interpretations of the political framework, based on the 1995 Dayton Accords, as well as efforts by Bosniak, Croat, and Serb leaders to maintain control over their political and ethnic fiefdoms, will continue to undermine Bosnia's central state institutions.[7]

As will be discussed in this chapter, these political, religious, economic, and ethnic disputes have adversely impacted the following:

The predicament of the more than two million refugees.

Further efforts to find the nearly 15,000 persons still missing and unaccounted for in 2015.[8]

Assistance to the surviving family members of the disappeared.

The effort to bring to justice the thousands of war criminals who still walk on the streets of the Bosnian war's battlegrounds.

The capacity of the post-1995 Bosnian government to overcome its dysfunction without "a set of bold reforms" to the Constitution and its dual entity structure.[9]

"All That Dayton Peace Nonsense": Continuing Ethnic Mistrust and Hatred in Bosnia

On November 21, 1995, after three weeks of intense negotiations at the American Air Force Base in Dayton, Ohio, the four-year Balkan wars ended.[10] Signed by the parties in Paris on December 14, 1995, the Accords took effect immediately. Within a week, NATO-led IFOR troops, ultimately totaling sixty thousand, were on the ground in Bosnia, including twenty thousand American military, replacing the UNPRO-FOR troops. Their mandate: to insure that the warring factions did not return to open warfare. In December 2004 an EU peacekeeping force replaced NATO military. In 2015 there are about twelve hundred troops and under three hundred members of the International Police Task Force still trying to secure order and safety in the entire country.

The Dayton Peace Accords, December 1995, Annex 2, delineated the Inter-Entity Boundary Line between the two 1992–1995 entities: the Federation (Croat/Bosniak) and the Republika Srpska (Bosnian Serb). In Annex 4, the newly established nation of Bosnia-Herzegovina, with a population of almost four million, 46 percent Muslim, 38 percent Serb, and 15 percent Croat, retained the two entities.

The Bosnian Serb Republika Srpska formally received 49 percent of the territory, a net gain of 3 percent controlled by the entity; and the Muslim/Croat Federation of Bosnia-Herzegovina retained 51 percent of the pre-1992 territory. The new nation had a parliament, a state judicial system, and a three-person (a Serb, a Muslim, and a Croat) "hydra-headed presidency."[11] Bosnia's weak central government, and the two-chamber legislature, was responsible for foreign policy, law enforcement, air traffic control, and communications. The Annex also created a Central Bank and unitary monetary system. It established ten cantons (counties), 142 municipalities, and one district—the city of Brcko.[12]

Annex 4 contained the new Constitution for Bosnia. American lawyers, working closely with Ambassador Richard Holbrooke and Secretary of State Warren Christopher, drafted it.[13] It provided for the protection of human rights and the free movement of people, goods, capital, and services throughout the country. The Constitution established a federal-type constitutional state, not a confederation. The two entities could not secede from Bosnia.

All persons indicted by the ICTY or serving a sentence imposed by the ICTY were barred from running for office or holding any other appointive or public office. Additionally, the three Bosnian governments "pledged to cooperate with the tribunal, but are not explicitly required to arrest indicted people."[14]

The byzantine governance configuration laid out in the 1995 Peace Accords, moreover, was seen by the Americans as a transitory one. According to Ambassador Kornblum, its "complex mechanisms . . . were supposed to be replaced in three years with a more streamlined structure."[15] This has not occurred because of a fundamental disagreement "between the Bosniak leaders' desire for a unified state, which the Serbs and Croats will not allow."[16]

Both entities have their own legislatures. The UN's Office

Bosnia Governmental Organization Chart

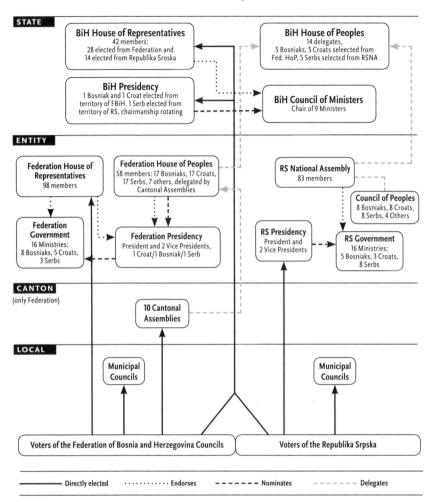

International Crisis Group (ICG), "Federation of Bosnia Herzegovina—A Parallel Crisis," *Relief Web Europe Report No. 209*, September 28, 2010, p. 26, at www.reliefweb.int/node/369534.

of High Commissioner for Human Rights (OHCHR) was charged with the task of civil implementation of the peace agreement.

Under Dayton's terms, Bosnian Serbs had to surrender suburbs of Sarajevo to the Federation, which also received some other eastern Bosnian areas held by the Serbs. Sarajevo became the capital of Bosnia-Herzegovina. In total, the 1995 Dayton agreement rearranged only slightly the pre-Dayton ethnic composition of the two entities.

In the Republika Srpska, almost 90 percent of the territory was formerly under the military control of the Bosnian Serbs, while Bosnian Croats had once occupied 9 percent, and little more than 1 percent was previously held by Bosniaks. The Federation, after the signing of the peace agreement, maintained 53 percent of territory formerly ruled by Bosniaks, 41 percent of territory once held by Bosnian Croats, and 6 percent of territory that Bosnian Serb forces subjugated before Dayton.[17]

A major problem the agreement attempted to deal with was the predicament of the more than two million refugees—both those internally displaced due to ethnic cleansing and the hundreds of thousands of refugees, mostly Muslim, "still in nearby countries like Germany, Austria, Switzerland, and Sweden."[18] The war and the ethnic cleansing that routinely occurred created a degree of chaos not seen in Europe since the end of the Second World War.

In Annex 7 of the Dayton Accords, all refugees and displaced persons could legally reclaim their homes or receive compensation. A Commission for Displaced Persons and Refugees was established to resolve conflicts regarding the return of property or the amount of compensation. It was authorized to issue final decisions. All persons living in Bosnia were granted the right to move freely throughout the country. In addition, the two entities were committed to cooperate with the ICRC in finding *all* missing persons.[19]

STARK REALITIES

However, the freedom of return, from the very beginning of the postwar era to the present, has had to confront the reality of continuing and, more ominously, escalating ethnic animosity between Bosnian Serbs, Muslims, and Croats. Just months after the Dayton agreement was signed, "even buses run by the UNHCR, designed to protect refugees visiting their old homes, have been stoned and many turned back."[20]

In summoning the parties to Dayton in late 1995, American president Bill Clinton said, "No one can guarantee that Muslims, Croats, and Serbs in Bosnia can come together and stay together as free citizens in a united country sharing a common destiny. Only the Bosnian people can do that."[21] However, two decades later, in Bosnia Herzegovina, this has not occurred. Furthermore, the prospect of the three ethnic communities "coming together" is very bleak.

From the very beginning of the post-1990s war era, there were harsh criticisms of the peace pact. First, coerced into accepting the Accords, the three ethnic communities almost immediately denounced the treaty's unfairness. The Bosnian Serbs, then and now, want a separate sovereign nation. Presidents of the RS have continually called for the establishment of an autonomous RS. On January 14, 2014, the latest missive came from Milorad Dodik. The RS president spoke on the twenty-second anniversary of the entity's founding. Before a distinguished group of Bosnian Serb leaders—government, clergy, and local officials—in Banja Luka, he reaffirmed the central axiom of the RS: autonomy and independence. "We are a state-building nation, which does not build a state for the sake of a state, but as a guarantee of freedom and development."[22]

The Croats were angry, then and now, because a separate Bosnian Croat entity was not established. The Bosniaks were angry, then and now, because the perpetrators of the war, who raped and committed war crimes, genocide, and crimes against humanity—the Bosnian Serbs—were *rewarded* under the terms of the Dayton Peace Accords.

Eric Stover put the dilemma in perspective in a 1999 interview: "The ethnic tensions and divisions in Bosnia are stronger now than they ever were before the war, because the war created them. In addition, part of the problem is the logic of politics,[23] which are based on ethnicity. [As] the system is structured now, a Croat votes for a Croat, a Serb for a Serb, a Muslim for a Muslim. Until you break that logic of politics now, you are going to continue to harden people's attitudes."[24]

Matters have not improved since 1999. On the tenth anniversary of the Dayton Accords, 2005, disapproval of them was near universal. Julie Mertus's essay reflected the views of the critics. She agreed with Stover's earlier assessment of the terrible ethnic politics at play in the nation. From the very beginning, she wrote, the Accords "was roundly criticized for rewarding the aggressor and cementing ethnic tensions into the architecture of the new state."[25]

The Accords "partitioned the country into two largely autonomous entities along ethnic lines, with a flimsy central government created which was to hold the complicated arrangement together." Mertus continues,

> The fear that the Dayton Accords would intensify ethnic divides has proven to be well founded. One-half the country is [seen] as a Muslim state, and the other half is regarded as the Serb state. Croats, who comprise 17% of the population, have no state. The election of stridently nationalist leaders remains common throughout the country. . . . Police often blatantly favor people from their own ethnic group, and Bosnian officials continue to refuse to cooperate fully with international efforts to try war criminals.[26]

There was, in 2005, a near-total lack of transparency in politics. The dilemma remains in 2015. Bosnia regularly appears on lists of *most corrupt countries.* "In a recent BBC poll, 97% of Bosnian citizens viewed their government as corrupt. . . . The rule of law often takes a back seat to the rule of force."[27] The problem of the refugees existed in 2005 and, in 2015, remains still unresolved. It is a reflection of the continued ethnic hostility in the nation. "Hundreds of thousands of displaced people still cannot return home safely. People returning home to a situation where they are now ethnic minorities face violence, harassment, and discrimination."[28] If in 2005 the country was described as a "troubled, ethnically divided state,"[29] the view a decade later has not improved. The High Representative of the EU in the country, Valentin Inzko, said: "The leaders of the three main ethnic groups still do not agree on what kind of country Bosnia should be, and the past several years have seen both major and mundane reforms put on hold because consensus cannot be reached. On this anniversary, we remember that peace is achieved by building *consensus* around areas of shared interest and *compromising* for the common good. I encourage Bosnia and Herzegovina's newly elected leaders to reflect on these issues . . . in order for their country to progress."[30] (my emphasis)

Valentin Inzko was still the EU's high commissioner when, in late October 2013, he was brought into another clash between the three ethnic groups. This still-unresolved controversy focused on the education of the young in the new nation. In Bosnia, there exist three school curricula implemented at the entity level: two (Croatian and Bosniak) in the Federation and one in the RS. All three have a common math and science curriculum (chemistry and biology), but all three have significant curricula differences in the "national" subjects: history, geography, religion, language and literature, and nature and society.

The incident Inzko confronted is a microcosm of the

chronic difficulty in the nation: the inability of the three groups to live agreeably, side by side, throughout the nation. In the eastern RS village of Konjevic Polje (close to Srebrenica), with a Bosniak majority, the primary school had 150 students—all Bosniaks. The main campus of the school, the Petar Kocic Primary, was located in the village of Kravice, populated mostly by Serbs. The school had ninety students, all Serbs. *All* schools in the RS are administered by the Education Ministry, with implementation of its policies by local officials. The local bureaucrats look after the curriculum, hire the faculty, and maintain the grounds and buildings across the region.

Initially, Bosniak parents complained to the ministry about the poor condition of the school building (no water, no working toilets, doors missing). Nothing was done by the RS officials to alleviate the situation. The parents escalated their criticism, alleging general discrimination, specifically, the inability of their children to learn "their" Bosnian language and study its literature. Further compounding the crisis were the dicta issued by the officials: unless their children attended Serbian language and literature classes, they would be expelled from school. The ethnic tensions in the area rose dramatically.

The Bosniak parents took their case to the street, setting up a tent city in Sarajevo, Bosnia's capital, across the street from the EU's Office of the High Commissioner, Valentin Inzko. Not only did the RS Education Ministry officials not take any action to solve the problem, they refused to engage in talks with the Bosniak parents. The protesting Bosniak parents said, "we seek protection from international institutions because authorities in Bosnia's mainly Serbian entity RS, offered no help. 'They have put us in a situation where we have to come here and demand our rights.'"[31]

However, Inzko, although consulting with the Bosniak group, had no solution to offer them. They had to negotiate with the RS Education Ministry. "The standpoint of the international community," said an OHC spokesperson, "is that the parents and the RS Education Minister need to get into direct contact again . . . because dialogue is the key to solution."[32] However, no meaningful conversation took place. To put an end to the crisis, in November 2013 Goran Mutabdzija, the RS Education Minister, announced that the entity will not renew the 2002 agreement it reached with the Federation, which "guarantees Bosniaks and Croats the right to be taught the five so-called national subjects separately." Beginning in September 2014, except for "mother tongue and religion," *all* primary school children in RS will follow the Serbian curriculum.[33]

This classic "catch-22" situation is the norm in Bosnia-Herzegovina. And that does not bode well for the nation. A Bosnian journalist gravely wrote: "An escalation in inflammatory political rhetoric has very possibly created a situation today in which *an isolated act of violence*, spontaneous or planned, could irreversibly destabilize Bosnia and Herzegovina."[34] (my emphasis)

The Possibility of Bosnia's "Irreversible Destabilization"

In 2011 two reports, by the U.S. Congressional Research Service (CRS) and by an international NGO, Amnesty International (AI), addressed the political and ethnic realities in Bosnia. Both were extremely critical of the lack of progress in the nation sixteen years after Dayton.

The CRS report's first paragraph set the tone of the document.

> Many analysts have expressed concern that the international community's efforts over the past 15 years to stabilize Bosnia are failing. Milorad Dodik, president of RS . . . has obstructed efforts to make Bosnia's central government more effective. He has repeatedly asserted the RS's right to secede from Bos-

nia. . . . Ethnic Croat leaders in Bosnia have called for the creation of a third, Croat "Entity," threatening a further fragmentation of the country. After two major Croat parties were excluded from the government of the Federation, they refused to recognize its legitimacy and formed their own assembly. . . . The combination of internal tensions within Bosnia and a declining international role could perhaps lead to violence and the destabilization of the region as a whole.[35]

The AI Annual Report 2011—Bosnia and Herzegovina was equally stark and pessimistic. "Relations between the [three] main ethnic groups continued to be marked by nationalistic rhetoric."

The *"Background"* section continued: "Continuous calls for separation by several high level politicians in RS threatened the stability of the country. On some occasions, Croat politicians also proposed the creation of a Croat-dominated Entity within Bosnia. In July, just before the 15th anniversary of the genocide at Srebrenica, several high level politicians of RS made statements *glorifying the perpetrators of this crime* . . . . Some of them denied the fact that genocide had taken place in Srebrenica.[36] (my emphasis)

An additional political nightmare that is looming is the near "ungovernability" of the Federation of Bosnia Herzegovina *itself* because of the continuing political clashes between Bosniaks and Croats in the entity. While these reports criticize the turbulent relationship *between* the Federation and the RS, there is "a parallel crisis *within* the Federation." Disputes among and between Bosniak and Croat leaders and a dysfunctional administrative system have paralyzed decision making, put the entity on the verge of bankruptcy, and triggered social unrest[37] (my emphasis).

On another major issue, the AI report indicated that survivors of rape and other sexually violent war crimes "continued to be denied access to economic and social rights

[and] live in poverty. They were unable to find work as they still suffered from the physical and psychological consequences of their war-time experience."[38] There was, because the government did not support psychological support for these survivors, very "limited" help provided to the victims by overburdened humanitarian NGOs. Although tens of thousands of women were sexually abused during the war, fewer than "2,000 women survivors of war crimes of sexual violence were receiving social benefits in the country based on their status of civilian victims of war."[39]

The AI report also noted the heightened discrimination in Bosnia and Herzegovina.[40] Roma and Jews continued to be denied the right to be elected to public office because they were not members of one of the three main ethnic/religious groups. (The Dayton Accords restricted this right to Bosniaks, Croats, and Serbs.) In December 2009 the European Court of Human Rights ruled that the constitutional framework and the electoral system discriminated against two plaintiffs (a Romani man and a Jewish man), and the state authorities were "obliged to amend it. The authorities failed to implement the judgment . . . [and] political attempts to change the constitutional framework, the electoral system and to reform the state institutions failed."[41] This ruling, through 2014, has not yet been implemented.

The AI report was very critical about the very "slow progress in identifying the whereabouts of victims of enforced disappearance during the war. . . . The whereabouts of between 10,000 and 11,500 people remained unknown."

Furthermore, because of the "inadequate response of the justice system, those responsible [for war crimes] often enjoy impunity."[42] Every report that examines the continued feasibility of the Dayton Peace Accords notes the heartless irony of victims and killers living next to each other. In the second decade of the twenty-first century, there has been an incremental increase in the number of individuals indicted and tried in Bosnian state courts for war crimes, rape, and genocide. While most charged are Bosnian Serbs, there has also been a small number of Croats and Bosniaks charged with war crimes. Some have been extradited from other nations, others arrested even though they held important law enforcement positions.[43]

With the ICTY not hearing new cases after 2014, *all* criminal proceedings will henceforth occur only in Bosnia-Herzegovina's state and entity courts.

An additional failing of the "state authorities [was their unwillingness and their inability] to create a database of the missing people and implement the Fund for the Support to the Families of Missing Persons—both of which were envisaged by the Law on Missing Persons (LMP) adopted in 2004."[44]

Anes Alic is a Bosnian political analyst who is quite skeptical about the nation's future. Unless there is *compromise and consensus* on the issues confronting the society, the future is bleak. "Republika Srpska officials will without any compromise stay the course of attempting to diminish the power of state institutions, and hints of secession will continue to circulate. Bosnian Croats will continue to work toward the creation of a third entity in the country, with a Bosnian Croat majority, under the perception that their ethnic identity is under threat. Bosniaks will continue to fight both."[45]

In his annual report to the UN Security Council in November 2013, Valentin Inzko, the high commissioner, soberly described the "challenges to the sovereignty and territorial integrity of the country, noting calls by senior officials in the RS for the dissolution of the country. [He said:] The RS President remains the most frequent and vocal critic of Bosnia's territorial integrity and sovereignty, recently boasting again that he will lead the entity to independence."[46]

Both entities were criticized by Inzko, who alluded to

the education crisis in the RS primary school system in his report. The problem was, in part, the consequence of the return to their homes of Bosniak refugees two decades after forced departures. The primary school crisis, he said, "reveals the failure of the competent authorities in Bosnia in the past 11 years to find a permanent, countrywide solution which would guarantee children's equal rights to education."[47]

There is, however, another festering problem, one that has been a less visible drama than the well-publicized bitter ethnic divisions championed by the ethno-nationalist political leaders since 1995. A huge disconnect has emerged since Dayton between the politicians in both entities and the general public. Because of the politicians' drive to acquire and maintain power—using all means to reach this end—while simultaneously ignoring the devastated economic condition of the nation, Bosnia's unemployment is one of the worst in all of Europe and is growing more dismal by the day.

In the second decade of the twenty-first century, Bosnia scarcely has a heartbeat. It is "a devastated country economically."[48] Matters have gotten worse two decades after the 1995 Peace Accords. Estimates of overall unemployment in the country range from 27 percent to 40 percent.[49] Also, in 2015 as many as 70 percent of young adults, including the future elites of the nation—musicians, poets, artists, writers, entrepreneurs, college graduate students, and others—cannot find work in Bosnia. Sajida Tulic, a twenty-seven-year-old unemployed Sarajevo actress protesting the miserable conditions, told a reporter that life in Bosnia "is not a way of living. We want our dignity back."[50]

These societal problems proliferate, but there is no attention paid by the political leaders of both entities and the state to address and then to "fix" them. Government corruption—at the municipal, canton, entity, and state levels—is rampant. Because of the shameless corruption and continued nurturing of racial and ethnic hatred by the politicians and government media outlets,[51] foreign investors were and remain unwilling to invest capital in the nation. In addition to high unemployment, there is no health care for nearly half the country's population, and infant mortality is one of the highest in Europe. Matters came to a head early in February 2014.

The Bosnian Spring: The Nation's "Wake-Up Call," February 2014

On Tuesday, February 4, 2014, thousands of infuriated Bosnians, the vast majority living in the Muslim-Croat Federation, "took to the streets [to] protest against the political paralysis and economic stagnation that have engulfed one of Europe's poorest and most divided countries."[52] The protest marches, labeled the "Bosnian Spring" by the demonstrators, continued in major federation cities, "with bursts of violence in Sarajevo, in the northern city of Tuzla [where the demonstrations began], in Mostar in the south, and in Zenika in central Bosnia."[53]

More than ten thousand factory workers, unemployed Bosnians, war veterans, and others set fire to government buildings and burned cars in Tuzla. This industrial city of two hundred thousand was in the throes of a major economic dislocation: its unemployment rate—55 percent—is the highest in the nation. The average unemployment figures for the country in 2015 range from 30 percent to 40 percent. And 67 percent of Tuzla's young people can't find any work.[54]

As the demonstrations continued, younger once-middle-class students and unemployed graduates joined the widespread antigovernment protests. They vented their anger at the local politicians "whom they view as self-serving and corrupt." The demonstrators called these officials "criminals," urging them to "resign today."[55]

Their call from the streets was a fundamental cry of desperation: "we want a new government of the expert, the young, and, above all, the uncorrupt."[56] The protesters had three essential demands: police must allow peaceful protests, and cantonal authorities "must guarantee security for all participants" in the protests; the people must decide on the formation of the next government; and "We seek the immediate resignation of the entire Federation government, starting with the Prime Minister."[57]

Hundreds were tear-gassed and injured during these actions; many were arrested and detained by the local police. A reporter spoke to an elderly man whose twenty-seven-year-old son had been taken by police in Sarajevo. Crying, he said that his son participated in the protests, that he did not know if his son had done anything wrong, "but he knew that, like many others, his son felt forced onto the streets because the conditions for people in Bosnia and Herzegovina today had become unbearable."[58]

Another observer on the scene said that Tuzla and Sarajevo looked like a "war zone. We haven't seen violent scenes like this since the war in the 1990s. People are fed up with what has become total political chaos in Bosnia, with infighting over power, a dire economic situation and a feeling that there is little hope for the future."[59]

Factory closings, along with unpaid salaries, pensions, and health benefits, triggered the Bosnian riots in Tuzla. Their rage quickly spread across the Muslim-Croat Federation (with only token support from citizens living in the RS). Some federation municipal and canton government officials resigned in the face of the rebels' anger.

Croatian and Serbian government leaders met with ethnic Bosnian officials in Tuzla (where ethnic Croatians are the majority) and in the RS (where ethnic Serbians control that entity) to try to "calm" the unrest and violence in Bosnia.[60] RS leaders, including President Dodik, insisted "that the protesters are overwhelmingly Bosniak and that the protests are aimed at destabilizing Republika Srpska."[61]

According to analysts, paralleling the emergence of the "Arab Spring," social media—especially Twitter and Facebook—played a major role in "harnessing long-simmering frustration and anger at state corruption" in Bosnia.[62] For the first time, one blogger wrote, "politicians became afraid of citizens, an observation made by many on Facebook and Twitter as cantonal governments resigned and some reportedly even left the country."[63]

Thus far in 2015, it is too early to tell the eventual outcome of the Bosnian Spring demonstrations. There has been silence from the European Community and from the U.S. State Department. Bosnia's future is, at this moment, tottering on the brink of dissolution. In all this turmoil, the issue of finding and identifying the dead and the causes of death still awaits further work by the forensics teams in Bosnia's killing fields.

The Impact of the "Bosnian Spring" on Finding the Disappeared and Helping the Survivors of the Missing

How have these "unprecedented levels of gloom about the future of the country,"[64] highlighted by the emergence of the Bosnian Spring, affected the difficult task of finding the graves and identifying the human remains? Whatever the final outcome of the nation's furious demonstrations and demands by frustrated Bosnians for significant changes in the character of government, there remains a serious, adverse impact on those tasked with finding and identifying the disappeared. In addition, the many tens of thousands of surviving family members who wait for the truth about the fate of their loved ones continue to suffer and live in a tragic twilight zone while the nation struggles to survive.

During the wars in Bosnia, 1991–1995, more than one hundred thousand people were killed, nearly 2.5 million others were displaced, and tens of thousands of people disappeared. It is nearly impossible to determine the precise numbers of those disappeared because of politically motivated *misinformation* from the three ethnic groups. Bosniaks, Bosnian Croats, and Bosnian Serbs alike minimize the number of enemy missing and enlarge the numbers of their own missing.

Bosnian Serbs still deny that their military violated the laws of war, especially the crime of genocide. Twenty-first-century Bosnian Serb partisans have gone as far as to delete the word genocide from a Bosniak Memorial in Visegrad in 2014 because of "the problem we have" with that word. (The Bosnian Serb municipal authorities, escorted by police, entered the Muslim cemetery before any Bosniak mourners arrived and erased the word from a memorial plaque because it was "offensive" to the locals.) Although ICTY guilty verdicts were handed down for "crimes against humanity" in the Visegrad area, there were no "genocide" convictions of perpetrators from Visegrad itself, although a number of defendants were convicted of genocide against Bosniaks in other killing zones, especially the Srebrenica area, during the 1992–1995 war.[65]

A culture of denial continues to exist across the paralyzed nation. "Everyone protects their 'own' criminals," wrote one observer of this omnipresent phenomenon.[66] In 2010 the UN Working Group on Enforced or Involuntary Disappearances (WGEID) wrote, after visiting Bosnia, "the number of missing persons is a highly political and controversial issue. There are disagreements about the number of people who went missing." In late 2010 the WGEID concluded that between twenty-eight thousand and thirty thousand people disappeared. The group estimated about two-thirds of the people have been accounted for, while one-third remain missing.[67] However, in February 2012, the ICMP and the ICRC concluded, after reviewing thirteen different sources, that the total number of missing in the Bosnian war was thirty-five thousand, most of them Bosniaks.[68]

All observers of the ethnic prejudice and massive government corruption in Bosnia since 1995 despair over its terrible impact on the agencies responsible for finding and identifying the disappeared, helping the survivors with financial and medical assistance, and punishing the perpetrators of war crimes and genocide. The UN Human Rights Council, the UN's WGEID, the European Union, global NGOs such as Amnesty International, Track Impunity Always (Trial), Physicians for Human Rights, as well as Bosnian humanitarian NGOs,[69] have published reports and provided testimony condemning the lack of progress.

In November 2004 the Law on Missing Persons went into force in Bosnia. It was written to safeguard the rights of the families of the missing in the new state. There are a number of key articles in the statute that affect the status of the missing and their families. They have not been adequately implemented and, given the 2014 Bosnian Spring antigovernment demonstrations, they will continue to founder.

The following three articles are crucial for the full implementation of the protocols for finding the disappeared and helping the survivors:

Article 7 of the LMP calls for the *creation* of a statewide organization to find and identify the missing, the MPI.

Article 15 requires the state to establish and fund a Fund for Support to the Families of Missing Persons.

Article 21 obliges the *immediate* establishment of a statewide central data bank of information about *all* the missing for utilization by the MPI.

The 2004 LMP was a major effort to deal with the profound problems associated with the disappeared. When the three primary articles were implemented, there would exist a central organization for finding and identifying the missing, a central database used by the MPI, as well as timely assistance—financial and medical—for the surviving family members of the missing.

However, by the time of the Bosnian Spring, major implementation deficiencies left the problems relating to the disappeared largely unresolved. These are the *ineffective* functioning of the MPI, the *nonestablishment* of an accurate and complete Central Records of Missing Persons (CEN) by Bosnian authorities, and the *absence* of a Fund for Support to the Families of Missing Persons.[70]

The Compromised Functioning of the MPI

There are a number of serious obstacles to the successful functioning of the MPI. Vacancies on the steering committee have not been filled by the state due to political distrust by the ethnic groups as well as the unwillingness of the governing elites to compromise and share power with their opposition. Operating budgets for 2011 and 2012 were seriously delayed because of the inability of the entities' leaders to form a government nearly two years after elections. These are serious organizational problems that delay the effective functioning of the MPI.

A more serious problem, one that goes against the *raison d'être* of the MPI, is the departure, five months after the MPI began fully functioning in 2008, of RS representatives from the MPI and the simultaneous creation of the RS Operative Team for Missing Persons. This parallel organization collects data relating *only* to missing Bosnian Serbs in Bosnia.

On the official website of the new RS search group, the government explained its break with the MPI: "Because of the dissatisfaction of family's [sic] of missing persons from the Republic of RS about the work of the [MPI] . . . , [and] the lack of results finding missing Serbs, . . . the Government of RS, on June 6, 2008, on the request of family's [sic] made a decision to form the Operational Team of the Republic of RS for Tracking Missing Persons (RSOT). Therefore the [team] was formed to speed up the process of finding missing persons."

The RS government, "respecting the [2004] law about missing persons, defined the jobs and tasks of the Operational Team, and its jurisdiction that is harmonized with the law for missing persons." The government pledged that the actions of the new organization "do not supersede the work of the MPI, but help it operate."[71]

However, as repeated cables to U.S. intelligence and national security agencies point out, "despite promises by RS prime minister Milorad Dodik that the RSOT would work cooperatively with MPI, practically the opposite has happened." MPI property has been confiscated by RSOT; MPI workers have been denied access to its offices, archives, and morgues in the RS as prosecutors refused to cooperate with MPI. And, in a spiteful catch-22, RS criticism of MPI work has increased because "[MPI] is not doing its job."[72]

These serious disagreements rage on in the press and on the airwaves. For example, in February 2011, war victims associations in RS blasted the leaders of the MPI, claiming that the organization did not do enough to find missing Bosnian Serbs. Of 702 mortal remains identified in 2010, only 32 were Bosnian Serbs (even though the majority of the missing in the 1992–1995 war are Bosniaks). "The associations in the RS refuse to accept that because this is not in line with what the RS officials have been saying," commented a political analyst to a reporter.[73]

It is understandable that collaboration between the MPI and the RS group is virtually nonexistent; and this reality has "fostered a climate of distrust, overall confusion, and animosity." For example, the director of the RS Missing Persons Team "often releases statements to the press that underestimate the work of the MPI and that question the official numbers and figures of missing Bosniaks in Bosnia."[74]

This rancor leads to conflicts between the two groups in the exhumation process itself. Before a gravesite is exhumed and the mortal remains are identified, it is necessary to get a court order. The lack of communication between the two groups slows down this process. By law, the MPI is the only organization that transmits possible gravesite locations to the state prosecutor who, in turn, asks the court to issue the exhumation permit. If the RS team's information is not given to the MPI, the finding and identification of the missing is delayed. This delay cruelly continues the pain and suffering of the surviving family members.

The law pertaining to the exhumation process itself is "complicated and subject to problems." Getting a court order for exhumation "has not always been easy, and determining which court and which prosecutor has jurisdiction has been a complicating factor," concluded the WGEID. (The process has changed: after January 2011 *all* exhumations and identifications became the responsibility of the State Prosecutor's Office.)

Further muddying the process is the fact that there are not enough prosecutors working on exhumation and identification. "Additional staff should be appointed to accelerate the process," concluded one reviewing agency of the UN. However, funding for the work has been cut in recent years. This lack of personnel slows the process and the anguish of the families continues.

Still another ongoing exhumation dilemma the MPI has not been able to resolve is that some of its field operations are below international forensic standards in the manner, quality, speed, and transparency of the process. The lab facilities need upgrading; there are not enough forensic pathologists and anthropologists. There is also a paucity of psychotherapists to assist the survivors of the war and the families waiting to hear about their missing family members. The state has not yet created a comprehensive program for all who need this medical assistance.

Another basic exhumation quandary still exists in the devastated nation. The receipt of information regarding the whereabouts of the gravesites *must* precede the exhumation and identification activities. That critically important information has become harder to obtain two decades after the war ended. "It is perpetrators who largely have the information on where graves could be found. Thus, it is important to bring perpetrators to justice to try to enhance the truth discovery process."[75]

This means that the perpetrators must be prevailed upon by the MPI and prosecutors to provide this information. This is extremely difficult for a number of reasons. Some merciless perpetuators "who know about mass graves are asking for money from families in order to reveal where the burial sites are." Others are fearful that revealing such information will label them as "traitors" in their ethnic community. To overcome such realities and have people reveal the critical information, the WGEID recommended that "witness protection programs be strengthened."[76]

Another distressing issue concerns how to balance the need to bring the perpetuators of these crimes to justice versus the need to bargain with them to get gravesite locations. In Bosnia in 2015 these alleged criminals continue to "live side by side with their victims, due to their large number, believed to be in the thousands, making it almost impossible to try them all in a short period of time." Essentially, continued secrecy and impunity remains a problem in the country and makes the discovery of the location of the graves of the more than eleven thousand undiscovered disappeared very problematical.

The conscience-stricken former soldier does, however,

STARK REALITIES

still exist and does, albeit more infrequently, reveal the whereabouts of these missing gravesites. In August 2013, for example, a Bosnian Serb military veteran anonymously "tipped off" the authorities about the location of a mass gravesite in northeastern Bosnia, near the town of Prijedor (one of the locations named in the genocide indictments handed down against Karadzic and Mladic, the leaders of the Bosnian Serb government during the war).[77]

The Bosnian State Prosecutor's Office immediately called for the exhumation of the site, which began in September 2013 and was scheduled to continue through the first part of 2014. The site contains the mortal remains of many hundreds of Bosniaks and Croatians murdered in the summer of 1992.

Thus far, the remains of nearly four hundred bodies have been found in graves often ten meters deep and located in no less than five scattered mass grave locations in the vicinity of Prijedor. The bodies are believed to be those of former civilian Muslim residents of the small villages and towns killed by Bosnian Serb soldiers "conducting house-to-house searches," then buried and reburied in these once-secret gravesites. The MPI believes the site "will turn out to be the largest mass grave from the 1992–1995 war, surpassing the 629 bodies found in [one mass grave in] Srebrenica."[78]

There are, in 2015, however, less than ten thousand persons missing nearly one-quarter century after they "disappeared."

The Long-drawn-out Establishment of the Central Record of the Missing Persons (CEN)

The CEN "intended to include all records that were or are kept at local or entity levels, by associations of families of missing persons, Tracing Offices of the organizations of the ICRC in Bosnia, as well as other international organizations." Article 22.4 of the LMP prescribed that the process of verifying and entering data in the CEN be accomplished by January 1, 2009.

In 2012 the CEN still "ha[d] not been completed or made public." Personnel and resources for the CEN were minimal. There were only six employees working on the completion of the CEN [and] it was not expected that the registry would be online and in use soon.

In the absence of any discernible movement to complete the task by entity administrators and politicians, the ICMP and the ICRC assumed the task and presented a working list of the missing to the MPI in late 2012.

The Lack of Agreement on Establishing the Fund for Support to the Families of Missing Persons

Article 15 of the LMP required the country to create a fund to assist the families of those who disappeared in the war. It called for the Council of Ministers to set up the fund "within 30 days from the date of the coming into force of the LMP [on November 17, 2004]." In 2012, more than seven years after the required deadline, the fund had not been established. Further, "there does not seem to be any significant development and Bosnian authorities do not show any willingness to address this matter." The dire situation still exists in 2015, and the survivors still cope with PTSD, other psychological illnesses, and the absence of closure.

There are two reasons for the interminable delay, and both reflect the political discord existing in the nation: the failure to agree on the location of the fund and the amount of money each entity should contribute to it. They have different views on which entity should pay a greater share. For the multiple thousands of surviving family members of the missing, a majority of them abused women and children, this ongoing stalemate produces a grim, sad result: the lack of social, medical, and financial support for the survivors.

A number of UN agencies and international NGOs have made recommendations to improve the nation's stability and to move along the complex process of identifying the missing and helping their families. In December 2010 the ICRC made three general suggestions:

1. Initiate an extensive search for gravesite locations and information on the fate of missing persons in the state's archives.

2. Speed up the identification of already exhumed bodies and provide increased resources to national commissions on missing persons and their forensic structures.

3. Exchange information *unconditionally* on the whereabouts of missing persons.[79] (my emphasis)

The UN's WGEID recommendations about the state of affairs in the country, placed before the UN General Assembly in late December 2010, addressed the problems brought about by the "increasingly compulsive politics and *irresponsibility* among local political elites."[80]

1. The families of the missing have the right to the truth about the progress and results of investigations conducted by the state and entity agencies.

2. The ICMP must remain actively engaged with forensic work in Bosnia.

3. The MPI must be supported and strengthened; its independence "should be guaranteed."

4. More resources and all available technology to detect graves and to exhume them must be made available to the MPI.

5. The MPI must be "provided with more political and financial support [and] supported to a greater extent by the RS authorities."[81]

6. Many more prosecutors are required to work on exhumations and war crimes prosecutions. More resources and support staff are also necessary. In January 2014, the European Union, in an effort to overcome some of these weaknesses, announced the allocation of 15.8 million euros to Bosnia for hiring judges, prosecutors, and additional staff members.

The official organ of the Bosnian government, the High Judicial and Prosecutorial Council of Bosnia, made the announcement: "The [EU] resources should become operational on February 15. The Project covers 16 prosecutors' offices and seven courts in Bosnia."[82]

The EU *had* to assist the government. Indeed, it is the first time that the organization ever "used this method of financing in a pre-[EU] accession country."[83]

7. More forensic scientists must be hired and provided with "needed assistance and equipment for exhumations."

8. Plea agreements with "persons suspected of having information on missing persons" must be continued.

9. The highest priority must be given to the fully funded establishment of the Fund to the Families of Missing Persons.[84]

These assessments and observations address both the political instability of Bosnia as well as the lack of financial commitment to continuing the complex and expensive process of finding, exhuming, identifying the missing, and assisting the families of the disappeared. It is problematic whether the authorities—at the national level and in the entities—have the political *will* to compromise and develop consensus on these issues. To this point, there is no evidence of such behavior on the part of the vast majority of state and entity politicians. The February 2014 Bosnian

Spring demonstrations put an exclamation point onto Bosnia's political spinelessness.

Until and unless there is such a significant substantive change in the behavior of the governing leaders across the nation, the plight of the missing and their families will continue. "Although victims should be in the focus when talking about [ending the problems], they are still forgotten and marginalized," said a representative of a local NGO, Citizens Committee for Human Rights. "We see no political will to compensate the victims," said another member of that NGO.[85] Furthermore, and sadly, most of the killers remain free, living with a high degree of impunity across Bosnia. Impunity is a reality that that will only increase as potential eyewitnesses age and die.[86]

The Power of History in Bosnia

Nick Hawton covered the events in the former Yugoslavia for the BBC for six years, 2002–2008, from Sarajevo and Belgrade. After his departure he wrote, "Like nowhere else I have visited, history lived and lives vividly in the minds of the people. The power of history or family or community folklore is overwhelming."[87] Wherever he traveled, he saw "historical labels" tacked on answers to his questions. For most, the 1992–1995 war "is a continuation of the Second World War, as if there had been just a short interlude between then and now. Some other Serbs I spoke to went further: strongly suggesting that the atrocities today were justified by the atrocities of the past. . . . If I spoke to a Croat or a Muslim about the conflict, the discussion would rapidly transform into a discussion about other conflicts in the last 50 years, or 200 years, or 500 years."[88]

After General Mladic was finally captured in 2011 and transported to The Hague to await trial before the ICTY, a *New York Times* reporter, Matthew Brunwasser, thought it was a turning point in the war against the "myths of which Balkan lore has so long been spun. For centuries here, history has been written in cycles of violence, reconciliation, new wars, exhaustion, and then more bloodshed. Each turn creates too much suffering to consume, and is grist for fresh lore to reinforce tribal instincts."[89]

However, Brunwasser included in his story a telling observation from the deputy mayor of Srebrenica, presently inhabited by Bosnian Serbs. Bosnia, the official told the *Times* reporter, still has "'three stories, three truths, and three histories' of the war: Serbian, Croatian, and Muslim."

Sadly, he pointed to the cruel reality in Srebrenica. The Srebrenica Peace Memorial Bosniak Cemetery and Museum attracts "school groups from Japan, America, and Europe, but not one group comes here from the Srebrenica School."[90] At literally the same moment, a Bosnian Serb living in Bratunac, a short distance from Srebrenica, told another reporter, "I have decided to frame a big photo of [General] Mladic and put it in my office, as a sign of respect for him, . . . and 99.9 percent of people in RS feel that way."[91]

This "power" of history holds sway on the population living in the former Yugoslavia and will determine the future of Bosnia. A defense attorney for many Serbs and Bosnian Serbs tried for war crimes and genocide at The Hague—including Radko Mladic—is convinced that the gap between the ethnic communities "remains so wide" that it cannot be bridged by guilty verdicts.[92]

There are very few persons and groups, aside from the NGOs representing the families of the missing, willing to address the potent hold of the past on the nation's future. To do so is to risk ostracism from one's community and even danger.

A telling example of this state of affairs: After a vote in the RS parliament that reflected this cultural and historical reality, one of the very few who *wanted to vote against the bill but did not* spoke to a reporter: "There was such an atmosphere around us that if we had voted against it, we would have been proclaimed enemies of the state. *We could not do a thing. So we ended up having no soul or morality. We ended up victims of paranoia in which people think that war criminals are at the same time heroes.*"[93]

On August 30, 2013, a small story in the *New York Times* underscored the terrible reality of life in Bosnia two decades after the horrors of refugee displacement, war crimes, rape, and genocide:[94] "Singing Serbian national songs and waving flags, [thousands of] people welcomed home as a national hero a convicted war criminal, Momcilo Krajisnik. Mr. Krajisnik, 68, was arrested and convicted by the [ICTY] of persecuting non-Serbians during the war in Bosnia from 1992 to 1995. A former speaker of the Bosnian Serb Parliament, he was granted early release from a British prison, where he had served two-thirds of a 20-year sentence. He flew to Banja Luka [in RS] and a government helicopter took him home to his wartime stronghold of Pale, near Sarajevo."

The acrimony between the three ethnic groups has not dissipated. It emerged—again—at the opening of the 2014 Winter Olympics in Sochi, Russia. A stalemate between the two Bosnian entities had rattled Bosnian Olympic officials. The issue: who will carry the nation's flag and lead the athletes marching into the stadium? Should it be Zana Novakovic, a skier from RS? Or should Igor Lajkert, a skier from the Federation, lead the parade? The rancor between the three Bosnian communities long ago ceased to surprise the population.[95]

Final Thoughts

Central to an explanation of the nation's citizens' dispirited mood and feelings of desperation is the total inability of Bosnia's political elites to even address the innumerable calamities—corruption, economic deterioration, and continual in-fighting among the three ethnic-political elites—much less resolve them. Unless there is a fundamental change in the Bosnian politicians' insistent commitment to "zero-sum ethnic politics," the society will be unable to end its downward spiral toward dissolution.[96]

Without change, Bosnia-Herzegovina will not move beyond its political, economic, and moral paralysis. Without such a needed dynamic change in Bosnia's all-or-nothing ethnic politics and the three existing—and clashing—views of history held by the politicians, the unraveling of the nation will proceed apace.

Much like the earlier failed Arab Spring, the 2014 Bosnian Spring demonstrations will probably not redirect the nation's prospect for change. The future is dismal. However, the festering boil has been pricked by the demonstrators. Most Bosnians, regardless of ethnicity, simply want a normal life in a country free of the politically cancerous corruption. A seventy-eight-year-old pensioner reflected the beliefs of his country's demonstrators: "I'm a Croat Catholic, but that is what I am at home. When I leave the house, I'm a citizen. I am sick and tired of this Serb, Croat, Bosniak. We have seven or 10 or however many levels of government and three presidents. We should have just one. Enough with this nationalism. But nobody is listening to me."[97]

. . .

In the meantime, the two-decade hunt for the "disappeared" continues—with all the attendant problems the forensic researchers still encounter. Especially galling to the survivors is vehement rejection, principally by Bosnian Serb political and military leaders (and other passionate RS residents), of the charge that genocide occurred in Bosnia. "Denial persists. The Serbs fund efforts to deny the Srebrenica slaughter. . . . They dream of statehood or union with Serbia."[98] The lack of any meaningful movement to address Bosnia's political gridlock and to deal with the location of the many still-undiscovered gravesites results from bitterness brought on by their assertions. "Genocide and its consequences are one of the fundamental reasons why our society is paralyzed, why such hatred is present, why we are still at war fought by different means."[99]

Recently, a group of forensic specialists, from the MPI and the ICMP, traveled to a small village in the RS. A few days earlier, a dam was shut down for repairs, lowering the water level of the Drina River. The low water revealed a number of skeletons believed to be missing Bosniak victims of the Visegrad violence in the first months of the Bosnian war.

Amor Masovic, one of the directors of the MPI, led the six-person group and, within a few days, they found two dozen additional mortal remains along the riverbank and in the Perucac Lake near Visegrad. As they left the boat, shots were fired at them. Masovic immediately reported the incident to the local RS police in Visegrad. The police told the media that the shots "were probably stray bullets from a hunter, not a murder attempt."

Masovic insisted that "it was a murder attempt," with one bullet missing him by no more than five centimeters.[100] The Bosnian Serb police never found the "hunter." However, the forensic investigators found more than 200 remains of the disappeared in the lake and, using DNA technology, have already identified 160 of the once-missing victims.[101] The ICMP reported, in October 2014, that there are still over nine thousand not accounted for. [102]

NOTES

Introduction

1. In July 2013, at the Mladic trial in the ICTY, a Danish demographer, Helge Brunborg, testifying for the prosecution, noted that the latest data showed 7,692 men missing after July 1995. The prosecutor then pointed out that "newer data" will be presented by other witnesses. Radosa Milutinovic, "7,692 Men Missing after July," *Justice Report*, July 25, 2013, at www.justice-report.com.

2. Emir Suljagic, "Truth at the Hague," *New York Times*, June 1, 2003.

3. Maass, *Love Thy Neighbor: A Story of War*, 39. Towns occupied by the Bosnian Serbs "became slaughterhouse[s]."

4. MacLean and Danziger, *Missing Lives*.

5. According to the ICRC, in 2010 there were 34,389 missing in Bosnia. Of that number, 19,168 were identified by forensic scientists. Still unaccounted for were more than 15,221 persons. See MacLean and Danziger, *Missing Lives*. Paul-Henri Arni, ICRC Director, Regional Affairs, Balkans, "Nearly 15,000 War Missing Still Haunt the Balkans," *Hurriyet Daily News and Economic Review*, August 29, 2010, at www.hurriet dailynews.com.

1. The "Disappeared" in War

Epigraph: Director, BIRN, Bosnia and Herzegovina Office, Sarajevo, Bosnia, July 4, 2014. A Bosniak survivor told her: "My children were killed, my wife was killed, my mother, my cousins. . . . They are not missing, they were killed. Their bodies are missing. I came back from Germany to find the bodies and because I want those responsible for what was done to be prosecuted," at www.balkaninsight.com.

1. Selma Ucanbarlic, "Families of the Missing Request Information about War Crimes," *Justice Report*, July 19, 2013, at www.justice -report.com.

2. Ucanbarlic, "First and Last Names Tell Us Who Perpetrated War Crimes, " *Justice Report*, July 26, 2013, at www.justice-report.com.

3. In Africa: Angola, Cote d'Ivore, Democratic Republic of the Congo, Eritrea, Ethiopia, Namibia, Somalia, Sudan, Zimbabwe. In Asia and the Pacific: Indonesia, Nepal, Pakistan, Philippines, Sri Lanka, Timor-Leste. In Europe: Armenia, Azerbaijan, Bosnia, Croatia, Cyprus, Georgia, Macedonia, Russian Federation, Serbia (Kosovo). In the Americas: Argentina, Chile, Colombia, Guatemala, Haiti, Peru. And in the Middle East and North Africa: Iran, Iraq, Jordan, Kuwait, Morocco, Syria.

4. Dusan Stojanovic, "World Marks Day of the Missing," August 29, 2012, at www.ap.org.

5. The first war, begun in 1991, involved Croatia, ethnic Croatians in Bosnia, and Serbia.

6. See *Srebrenica Genocide Blog*, "Bosnian Death Toll: 104,732 (Minimum)," at www.srebrenicagenocide.org.

7. This figure has changed over time. In 2008 the number of missing was placed at forty thousand persons. See ICMP report, June 2008, at www.ic-mp.org/. In 2010 the UN Office of the Commissioner of Human Rights issued a new number of disappeared: thirty-four thousand persons, with nearly thirty thousand disappeared in Bosnia during 1992–1995. More than twenty-seven thousand of the disappeared are Bosnian Muslim civilians. See www.commissioner.coe.int and www .iwpr.net/report-news/Bosnia-un/.

8. Some of the countries with missing persons include Chechnya, Cyprus, Sudan, Rwanda, Cambodia, Algeria, Nepal, the Philippines, Iraq, Chile, Guatemala, Colombia, Argentina, Congo, Kashmir, and East Timor. See Kathryne Bomburger, ICMP Director, Speech, July 2007, 3, at www.ic-mp.org/cos.63.1doc.

9. UN Commission on Human Rights, "Question of Enforced or Involuntary Disappearances," January 15, 1997, 4, at www.hri.ca/fortherecord1997 /documentation.

10. *Amnesty International Annual Report 2011–Bosnia*, May 13, 2011, at www.unhcr.org/refworld, 7. In 2015 the number of disappeared still not found remains less than ten thousand.

11. Quoted in MacLean and Danziger, *Missing Lives*, 58.

12. Brkic, *The Stone Fields*, 19.

13. Quoted in Sudetic, *Blood and Vengeance*, 353.

14. Pasagic, "Psychosocial Recovery in Bosnia-Herzegovina," 45.

15. See, for example, Quirk and Casco, "Stress Disorders of Families of the Disappeared," 1675–79.

16. Pasagic, "Psychosocial Recovery," 46.

17. Blaauw and Lahteenmaki, "Denial and Silence," 767.

18. Sassoli and Touga, "The ICRC and the Missing," 730.

19. Quoted in Mike O'Connor, "Muslim Widows in Bosnia Try to Rebuild Lives Without Men," *New York Times,* July 13, 1996, at www.pixelpress .org/Bosnia/context/.

20. O'Connor, "Muslim Widows in Bosnia."

21. O'Connor, "Muslim Widows in Bosnia."

22. O'Connor, "Muslim Widows in Bosnia."

23. O'Connor, "Muslim Widows in Bosnia."

24. In August 2004 William Haglund, director of the PHR forensics program, met with representatives from Cypriot and Turkish Cypriot communities "to discuss the exhumation of mass graves on the island of Cyprus. . . . The international community is urging Turkish and Greek leaders to continue to exhume the remains of both Turkish and Greek Cypriots." PHR *International Forensics Program,* "PHR Forensic Director to Cyprus to Discuss Exhumations," August 6, 2004, at www.phrusa .org/research/forensic/news_cyprus.html. The issue is still unresolved.

25. Pasagic, "Psychosocial Recovery in Bosnia-Herzegovina in the Aftermath of Violence," 47.

26. Herman, *Trauma and Recovery,* 4.

27. Courtney Angela Brkic, "The Wages of Denial," *New York Times,* July 11, 2005. Another Bosniak noted that, until one of the Serb defendants on trial at The Hague for crimes against humanity confessed to participating in Srebrenica's crimes, "I had never heard a Bosnian Serb admit that the massacre even happened." Suljagic, "Truth at The Hague."

28. Quoted in O'Connor, "Muslim Widows in Bosnia."

29. Selma Ucanbarlic, "Families of Missing Request Information about War Crimes," Balkan Investigative Reporting Network, March 2, 2012, at www.birn.eu.com.

30. The Argentine Forensic Anthropology Team (EAAF) was founded in 1984, with the help of Dr. Clyde Snow, an American forensic anthropologist, to investigate the disappearance of ten thousand Argentines during the 1976–83 military dictatorship.

31. In Iraq in 2003, CBS News reported that a mass grave, with two thousand bodies, was found in al-Hilla, south of Baghdad. "They died in terror. Many of the blindfolds were still in place." The ICMP forensic

team led the search. "As many as 300,000 mothers in Iraq live for the day they can bury their son. The loss in Iraq is 10 times greater than the Balkans." Scott Pelley, "Answers From the Grave," CBSNEWS.com, November 30, 2003, at www.cbsnews.com/stories/2003/11/26/60minutes.

32. Butolo, Maria, and Marion, *Life After Trauma*.

33. Quoted in Note, "Dole Will Help Identify Bosnia War Dead," *Orlando Sentinel*, August 29, 2000.

34. The Institute of Psychoanalysis, September 25, 2001, at www.psycho analysis.org/uk/goldstone.htm.

35. She said: "Survivors can really become victims when [their] expectations and hopes are raised. When you think that you have achieved a position where something will be done, some justice will be done, and yet many times over, because of political interests, nationalistic interests—whatever—these expectations and hopes are not fulfilled. Then, the survivors really become victims and they are betrayed and that is very, very dangerous for many people who have gone through that process. So we really must be very careful not to create expectations and then not fulfill them." The Institute of Psychoanalysis.

36. Pasagic, "Psychosocial Recovery in Bosnia-Herzegovina in the Aftermath of Violence," 46.

37. See generally Ball, *Prosecuting War Crimes and Genocide*, particularly chapter Seven, "The Rome Statute," 188–216.

38. The ICC is in its infancy and its prosecutors and judges are committed to cultivating the court's reputation as an even-handed, nonpartisan, permanent organization dedicated to providing justice to victims of major war crimes. Achieving acceptance as a court that dispenses justice evenhandedly is a very difficult task in the twenty-first-century fragmented world of *realpolitik* for a number of reasons, i.e., the mistrust of the ICC by one of the warring nations and the blind rage of many surviving victims of the cold-blooded crimes that fall under the ICC's jurisdiction that causes them to seek extrajudicial justice that the ICC cannot provide (the death penalty). There have been a very small number of cases heard by the ICC, most involving the dictators of small African nations. However, in September 2014, there emerged the possibility that the ICC would be asked to examine war crimes allegedly committed by a nation allied with the West, Israel. It was rumored that the ICC would be asked to hear a case involving a number of war crimes and crimes against humanity allegedly committed by Israeli military forces in the fifty-day summer 2014 war between Israel and Hamas in the Gaza Strip. Israel, one of less than ten nations who rejected the

1998 Treaty and has consistently maintained that the ICC is inherently political and biased against it, is unwilling to participate and, since it is not a signee, the issue would be moot. However, the Palestine Authority has threatened to join the ICC "for the purpose of holding Israel accountable for its actions [in Gaza]. The Court generally only investigates cases where the country involved is *unwilling* or *unable* to investigate itself." According to UN Human Rights Council (HRC, an agency severely biased against them, Israel leaders believe), reports, more than 2,100 Palestinians were killed in the Israeli air and ground actions, with "up to three-quarters of them civilians." Israel's Military Advocate General Corps, in an attempt to "pre-empt the impact of international inquiries into allegations of possible Israeli war crimes in Gaza," has ordered [its military] to conduct criminal investigations into a number of incidents." This is a potential situation fraught with danger for the ICC because of the duration and intensity of the hatred voiced by antagonists in this very unstable region of the world. See Isabel Kershner, "Israel Investigating Possible Gaza War Misconduct," *New York Times*, September 10, 2014, at www.nytimes.com.

39. Laura Shin, "The Science Behind Ratko Mladic's Trial," June 4, 2011, at www.smartplanet.com.

40. Clea Koff, interviewed on NOW, PBS, "International Justice," July 9, 2004, by David Brancaccio, at www.pbs.com.

41. Koff interview, NOW.

42. Koff, quoted in Shin, "The Science behind Mladic's Trial."

43. Koff interview, NOW.

44. DNA'S first use in the identification of the bones of Bosnian dead occurred in November 2001. Until then, forensic specialists working to identify the bones of the missing employed classic technology. DNA's use, as will be seen, has been *the* most important technological protocol in identifying the missing wherever forensics personnel are working in the world.

45. Stover and Peress, *The Graves*, 196–97.

2. Balkan Nationalism

Epigraphs: Quoted in *The Sun*, July 23, 2008, www.thesun.com.uk. Clark, *Sleepwalkers*, xxviii.

1. Malcolm, *Bosnia*, xix.

2. Six hundred years later, on the anniversary of the Serb defeat, Serbia's leader Slobodan Milosevic gave a speech commemorating the battle and called for the creation of a "Greater Serbia."

3. Malcolm, *Bosnia*, 51–53. "By the early sixteenth century several hundred thousand had probably converted. . . . The bishop of Zagreb wrote in 1536: 'More and more people are doing so [converting to Islam], hoping they will enjoy more peaceful times in what remains of their lives.'" Mazower, *The Balkans: A Short History*, 44, 46–47.

4. At the beginning of the 1991 wars in the former Yugoslavia, the Bosnian Muslims were 44 percent of the population (with 31 percent Bosnian Serbians and another 17 percent Bosnian Croats).

5. "Under Turkish rule, Jews found a haven and Eastern Orthodox believers were allowed to follow their religion." Sudetic, *Blood and Vengeance*, 10.

6. Sudetic, Blood and Vengeance, 49; Dedijer, *The Yugoslav Auschwitz and the Vatican*, 10.

7. Quoted in Maass, *Love Thy Neighbor*, 11. "Many potential frictions [between the groups], were blunted or diffused by shared local practices. Customs evolved to offer security and insurance across the religious divides." Mazower, *The Balkans*, 62. See also Heleta, *Not My Turn To Die*, 18: "My mom and dad refused to believe that people who had grown up together in peace and friendship . . . could overnight be blinded by ethnic hatred and start to kill one another."

8. Maass, *Love Thy Neighbor*, 69. "'Ethnic rivalry' was an erroneous term. . . . It was a mistake . . . to use 'ethnic' to describe the things that happened in Bosnia." Malcolm writes that "there is no such thing as a Bosnian face; there are dark-haired and fair-haired, olive-skinned and freckles, big-boned and wiry-limbed Bosnians. Bosnia is a human mosaic." Malcolm, *Bosnia*, xxiii.

9. Heleta, *Not My Turn To Die*, 18. During his criminal trial at The Hague, Radovan Karadzic argued that this reality was "caused by enormous hatred that was not only generated during that [1992–1995] war and the Second World War, but also during all other possible wars." Quoted in "Karadzic: Crimes Caused by Hatred," *Justice Report*, February 16, 2012, at www.birn.eu.com. The following day, Karadzic claimed the violence "happened according to a *historical automatism*." Quoted in "Karadzic: No Excuse for Murders," *Justice Report*, February 17, 2012, at www.birn.eu.com.

10. Maass, *Love Thy Neighbor*, 70.

11. This fourteenth-century Serb empire of Tsar Stepan Dusan was a huge territory comprising present-day Serbia, Albania, Macedonia, and central and northern Greece. Ironically, it did *not* include Bosnia.

12. Clark, *Sleepwalkers*, 19.

13. Hastings, *Catastrophe 1914*, 17.

14. Clark, *Sleepwalkers*, 21.

15. Clark, *Sleepwalkers*, 21–22.

16. Clark, *Sleepwalkers*, 22–23. "What was preserved above all within this tradition was the memory of the Serbian struggle against alien rule." (This was a reference to the Austrian-Hungarian and Ottoman empires.)

17. Sudetic, *Blood and Vengeance*, 14–15. Malcolm maintains that the Orthodox Church regularly "whipped up" Serb nationalistic attitudes. Malcolm, *Bosnia*, 171. Clark maintains that the Serbs' 1389 defeat at Kosovo Field "burgeoned into a symbolic set-piece between Serbdom and its infidel foe[s]." *Sleepwalkers*, 23.

18. Hastings drew parallels between these Serb terrorist groups and the IRA. "Serbians played something of the same violent role on the margin of the Hapsburg Empire as did Irish factions in the affairs of Britain at several periods of the twentieth century." Hastings, *Catastrophe 1914*, xxxii.

19. The action "roused Russian fury," wrote Hastings. Hastings, *Catastrophe 1914*, xxiv.

20. Clark, *Sleepwalkers*, 34–35.

21. When war began in 1914, the Serb military, initially, was surprisingly successful against the much larger Hapsburg forces. See Hastings, *Catastrophe 1914*, chapter Four, "Disaster on the Drina."

22. Clark, *Sleepwalkers*, 37.

23. Hastings, *Catastrophe 1914*, xxxiv.

24. The territory lost included Alsace Lorraine, captured by Germany in 1870, and returned to France; the German Saar, given to France for fifteen years, after which a plebiscite would determine the future of the region; Poland, which became an independent nation with a route to the sea that divided Germany in two; Danzig, a major German port, placed under international rule; all German and Turkish colonies, which were taken away and placed under Allied rule; Finland, Lithuania, and Czechoslovakia, which were made independent nations; and Austria-Hungary, split up, with a South Slav Kingdom, soon to be called Yugoslavia, being created. The Treaty of Versailles, signed June 28, 1919, was the document that changed the face of Europe for two decades. Millions of ethnic Germans lived in many of these newly created states, which led to unfortunate consequences for world peace in the mid- and late 1930s.

25. Malcolm, *Bosnia*, 171.

26. Matjaz Klemencic, "The Rise and Fall of Yugoslavia: From King Aleksandar to Marshall Tito, 1918–1980," in *The Slovenian*, 211–238, at www.slovenia.com. With the help of the Russians, Serbia became fully independent from the Ottoman Empire and a constitutional monarchy in 1878. Also, it was "the heart and soul of the pan-Slav movement." Hastings, *Catastrophe 1914*, xxx.

27. Klemencic, "Rise and Fall." In 1921 the kingdom's population was a little less than twelve million people. The four largest Slavic ethnic groups were Serbs (44 percent), Croats (24 percent), Slovenes (8.5 percent), and Muslims (6.3 percent). South Slavs mostly lived in four entities in the Balkan region—the Hapsburg Empire, Serbia, Montenegro, and Bulgaria—but under eight different government systems. "Their impassioned nationalism imposed a dreadful blood forfeit: about 16 per cent of the entire [Slavic] population, almost two million men, women, and children, perished violently in the six years of struggle [1912–1918]." Hastings, *Catastrophe 1914*, 16.

28. Klemencic, "Rise and Fall."

29. Klemencic, "Rise and Fall."

30. Ante Pavelic, 1889–1959, was born a short distance south of Sarajevo. After attending a Jesuit Seminary secondary school, he studied law at the University of Zagreb, in the capital of Croatia. He became a member of an extreme right-wing nationalist party that advocated freedom for Croatia. For Pavelic, the only reality was, as he wrote, "a free and independent Croat state comprising the entire historical and ethnic territory of the Croat people." Croatia's enemies, he said, were the Serbian government, international Freemasonry, Jews, and communists. In 1929 Pavelic came into contact with the new Italian dictator Benito Mussolini and, by 1932, relocated to Rome and turned the Croat Youth Movement into the notorious, dreaded Ustashe, a terrorist organization known for its hatred of Serbs and Bosnians. In 1934, while in France, the Yugoslavian king was assassinated by a small band of Ustashe terrorists. In 1934, Pavelic, still living in Italy, was tried in absentia for the royal assassination and sentenced to death by a French court. Italy refused to send Pavelic to France for his punishment. See Ball, *Genocide*, 124.

31. Klemencic, "Rise and Fall."

32. This 1939 boundary became viable when, in 1991, emissaries of Milosevic and Tudjman met in Austria to divide Bosnia between the two nations. See Bennett, "Izetbegovic."

33. Sudetic, *Blood and Vengeance*, 26. "The aim of the one-party Ustashe state was 'to work for the principle that the Croatian people alone will always rule in Croatia.'" Mazower, *The Balkans*, 123.

34. Malcolm, *Bosnia*, 176.

35. During World War II, the Ustashe used the phrase, "cleansing the terrain," to explain their brutal actions against the Serbs. Toal and Dahlman, *Bosnia Remade*, 3.

36. Sudetic, *Blood and Vengeance*, 26.

37. In Jasenovac, 750,000 Serbs were brutally exterminated along with 60,000 Jews and 26,000 Gypsies. Dedijer, *The Yugoslav Auschwitz*, 11.

38. Sudetic, *Blood and Vengeance*, 26–27.

39. Roy Gutman, *A Witness to Genocide*.

40. Klemencic, "Rise and Fall."

41. Klemencic, "Rise and Fall."

42. Tito was born in 1892. He was a soldier in the Austro-Hungarian Army and became a POW in Russia. In 1917 he became a Communist and joined the Red Army. He returned to Yugoslavia and became a leading Yugoslav Communist. He was imprisoned from 1928 to 1934 for Communist activities. Upon release, he resided in Moscow for a few years and, in 1937, he became secretary-general of the Yugoslav Communist Party. During World War II, he organized and led the Partisan Army against the Axis occupiers. After the war, he became the leader of the nation until his death in 1980.

43. Malcolm, *Bosnia*, 180.

44. Klemencic, "Rise and Fall."

45. See Davidson, "Death of Josip Broz Tito."

46. See David Bennett, "Alija Izetbegovic Biography," *Serendipity*, November 2000, at www.socialactionaustralia.org/2011/01.

47. Pavelic fled Croatia in 1945 for Rome, protected there by the Vatican. In 1948 he moved to a monastery near Rome, disguised as a Catholic priest. Later that year, Vatican agents smuggled him out of harm's way to Argentina, where he revived the Ustashe movement and served as an advisor to Argentinean president Juan Peron. Between 1946 and 1948, nearly eight thousand Ustashe veterans arrived in Argentina under Peron's protection. In 1957 the Yugoslavian secret police finally located Pavelic and planned his assassination. He was seriously wounded in the attempt and fled to fascist Spain, led by military dictator Francisco Franco. In 1959 Pavelic died from his wounds while living in Madrid. See Ball, *Genocide*.

48. Wagner, *To Know Where He Lies*, 191–92. Clark, too, notes that "the memory of the Serbian struggle against alien rule" repeatedly surfaced throughout the twentieth century. Clark, *Sleepwalkers*, 23.

49. Klemencic, "Rise and Fall."

50. Sudetic, *Blood and Vengeance*, 55.

51. Mazower, *The Balkans*, 140.

52. Bosnia-Herzegovina, at www.Atlapedia.com.

53. Klemencic, "Rise and Fall."

54. MacLean and Danziger, *Missing Lives*, 23.

55. Woodward, *Balkan Tragedy*.

56. Serbian Academy of Arts and Sciences, "Serbian Academy of Arts and Sciences (SANU) Memorandum, 1986, at www.chnm.gmu.edu/1989/items/show/674.

57. Courtney Angela Brkic, "Justice Denied in Bosnia," *Dissent* (Summer 2007), at www.dissentmagazine.org/articles.

58. Slobodan Milosevic, 1941–2006, was the first European head of state to be prosecuted for genocide and war crimes. From 1989 to 1999, while Serb president, he presided over mayhem and mass murder in Croatia, Bosnia, and Kosovo in the effort to create the "Greater Serbia." On November 23, 2001, Milosevic was charged by the International Criminal Tribunal for the former Yugoslavia (ICTY) prosecutor with the following crimes: "Genocide and complicity in Genocide; Crimes against humanity involving persecution, extermination, murder, imprisonment, torture, deportation and inhumane acts (forcible transfers); Grave breaches of the Geneva Conventions of 1949 involving willful killing, unlawful confinement, willfully causing great suffering, unlawful deportation or transfer, and extensive destruction and appropriation of property; Violations of the laws or customs of war involving *inter alia* attacks on civilians, unlawful destruction, plunder of property and cruel treatment." That he ended up in the dock in The Hague at all surprised many who watched his forceful behavior through the 1990s. He died at The Hague while his trial was in its fourth year.

59. Malcolm, *Bosnia*, 210.

60. Malcolm, *Bosnia*, 212.

61. Excerpts from his speech: "Six centuries later, now, we are being again engaged in battles and are facing battles. They are not armed battles, *although such things cannot be excluded yet*. However, regardless of what kind of battles they are, they cannot be won without resolve, bravery, and sacrifice, without the noble qualities that were present here in the field of Kosovo in the days past. . . . Let the memory of Kosovo heroism

live forever! Long live Serbia!" (my emphasis) at www.slobodan.milosevic
.org/spchKosovo1989.htm.

62. Sudetic, *Blood and Vengeance*, 78–80.

63. Norman Cigar wrote that Milosevic "brilliantly used the media to sell his ideology." *Genocide in Bosnia: The Policy of Ethnic Cleansing.*

64. Quoted in MacLean and Danziger, *Missing Lives*, 34.

65. Malcolm, *Bosnia*, 215.

66. Malcolm points out that, in 1990, Bosnian Muslims "were among the most secularized Muslim populations in the world." Malcolm, *Bosnia*, 221.

67. Tudjman was born on May 14, 1922, in Croatia, and died on Dec. 10, 1999, in Zagreb. He was a Croatian politician and president of Croatia (1990–99). He served with the partisans under Tito in World War II. Afterward, he stayed in the army and became a general. He taught political science and history at the University of Zagreb (1963–67) and later wrote numerous books on history and politics. In 1965–69, when he was a member of the Croatian parliament, Tudjman became increasingly nationalistic and in 1967 was expelled from the League of Communists and dismissed from his posts for nationalist "deviation." After the failure of the "Croatian Spring" of 1971, in which he had taken an active part, he was imprisoned for a year. After Tito's death in 1980 he became increasingly critical of the Communist political system and was again imprisoned for a year in 1981. In 1989 Tudjman founded the Croatian Democratic Union, which won Croatia's first free parliamentary elections in 1990. Named president, he pressed for the creation of a homogenous Croatian state, which became a reality in 1991. See Franjo Tudjman Biography, Bennett, at http://www.answers.com/topic/franjo-tudjman#ixzz1f2f728i1.

68. Alija Izetbegovic was born on August 8, 1925, and died on October 19, 2003. He grew up in Sarajevo and was a practicing Muslim all his life. During World War II, he joined the Young Muslims, an organization protected by the occupying Nazi forces. After the war, he was one of many thousands put on trial for his relationship with the Germans and was sentenced to three years in prison. Freed in 1947, he attended law school in Sarajevo. He practiced law and wrote philosophical treatises on the place of Islam in Yugoslavia and the world. In 1970, he published a controversial book, *The Islamic Declaration*, which advocated unity between Islamic teachings and culture. One could not be an ethnic Muslim and not be a believer. These ideas led, in 1983, to Izetbegovic once again being put on trial, this time accused of plotting to

establish an Islamic state. He spent five years in prison. Released in 1988, he founded the exclusively Muslim Party of Democratic Action, and the overwhelming majority of Muslims living in Bosnia (44 percent of 4.3 million people) supported "Dedo's" (Grandpa's) leadership of the party. In the November 1990 elections, he won the position of president of Bosnia and served in that position until 2000. Although unwilling to have Bosnia leave Yugoslavia and declare its independence, after Macedonia, Croatia, and Slovenia declared their independence, Izetbegovic had no choice. To remain in a truncated Yugoslavia meant domination by Milosevic's Serbian regime. Immediately after the February 29, 1992, successful vote for independence and the creation of the Republic of Bosnia-Herzegovina (1992–95), the war began with the siege of Sarajevo (which lasted three years). He governed a very splintered nation until his retirement in 2000. Three years later, after a fall, Izetbegovic died in Sarajevo. See David Bennett, "Alija Izetbegovic Biography," *Serendipity*, November 2000, at www.socialaction-australia.org/2011/01.

69. David Binder, "Alija Izetbegovic, Muslim Who Led Bosnia, Dies at 78," *New York Times*, October 20, 2003, at www.nytimes.com.

70. Sudetic, *Blood and Vengeance*, 82.

71. Quoted in Sudetic, *Blood and Vengeance*, 83–84.

72. Macedonia, one of the six republics in Yugoslavia, declared its independence at the same time, but that action was not followed by war because of the ethnic makeup of that territory. Slovenia declared its independence in 1991, and Milosevic accepted that action. There were few ethnic Serbs there, and it was an inhospitable region for warfare.

73. Dedijer, *Yugoslav Auschwitz*, 11–12.

74. Bosnia-Herzegovina, at www.Atlapedia.com. Reacting to Milosevic's tactic, Tudjman's armed forces attacked the ethnic Serb minority in Croatia, "driving them into Milosevic's hands" and triggering the start of hostilities. The ethnic Serbs, organized by the Yugoslav army, attacked Croatian forces, "thus beginning Milosevic's bid to dismember Croatia and create his own Greater Serbia." Sudetic, *Blood and Vengeance*, 81–82.

75. This phrase achieved worldwide notoriety when, in 1992, the second Bosnian War began between Bosniaks and indigenous Serb irregular armed forces, joined by Yugoslavian army troops and arms.

76. Sudetic, *Blood and Vengeance*, 87.

77. Mark Danner, "The U.S. and the Yugoslav Catastrophe," *New York Review of Books*, November 20, 1992.

78. Stover and Shigekane, "The Missing in the Aftermath of War," 848.

79. Koff, *The Bone Woman*, 194.

80. Koff, *The Bone Woman*, 211–12.

81. Franjo Tudjman, *Oxford Dictionary of Political Biography*, at http://www.answers.com/topic/franjo-tudjman#ixzz1f2pEwUi6.

82. Richard Holbrooke, *To End a War*, 21.

83. Adil Kulenovic, "Interview with Vladimir Srebov," *Vrebe*, Belgrade, October 30, 1995, in Danner, "America and the Bosnia Genocide."

84. Mladic's comments taken from minutes of May 12, 1992, meeting of the four Bosnian Serb leaders. Quoted in Marija Ristic, "Mladic 'Warned Bosnian Serb Leadership' About Genocide," *Balkan Transitional Justice*, September 20, 2013, at www.balkaninsight.com.

85. ICRC, Research and Documentation Center, *The Bosnian Book of the Dead*, June 21, 2007. www.srebrenicagenocide.org.

86. Quoted in Marc Danner, "America and the Bosnian Genocide," *New York Review of Books*, December 4, 1997.

87. Radovan Karadzic was born in Montenegro in 1945. His father, during World War II, was a Chetnik who fought the Ustashe and the Communist partisans. In 1960 he moved to Sarajevo, the capital of Bosnia, to study medicine. He graduated and worked as a psychiatrist until the demise of Yugoslavia in 1990. In 1992 Karadzic, SDP leader, proclaimed the formation of a Bosnian Serb Republic in Bosnia—Republika Srpska. After the war ended in 1995, both he and Radko Mladic were indicted for numerous crimes by the ICTY, which charged that the pair were "criminally responsible for the unlawful confinement, murder, rape, sexual assault, torture, beating, robbery and inhumane treatment of civilians." Thirteen years after the end of the war, in 2008, Karadzic was captured and turned over to the ICTY to answer the many charges against him. His trial has continued to the present time (2015).

Radko Mladic was born in Bosnia. The Ustashe killed his father in World War II. He entered the Yugoslav military and reached a command position in the 1970s. In 1991 he was appointed commander of the Ninth Corps of the Yugoslavian Army in Croatia. In 1992 he took command of the eighty thousand soldiers stationed in Bosnia. They immediately became the military backbone of the Bosnian Serb forces battling the Muslims and Croats in Bosnia. The notorious Bosnian Serb militias joined this force and, in less than two months in the spring of 1992, under his leadership, they seized control of 70 percent of the country. In late 2010 Mladic was finally apprehended and is still on trial at The Hague in 2015, charged with war crimes and genocide. Sudetic, *Blood and Vengeance*, 169.

88. Quoted in Sudetic, *Blood and Vengeance*, 86.

89. These units included the dreaded Red Berets, the Black Wolves, the Drina Wolves, the White Eagles, the Speciaina Policia, the Arkan Tigers, and Seslj Militia. See Mark Danner, "The Killing Fields of Bosnia," *New York Review of Books*, September 24, 1997.

90. Mark Danner, "Bosnia: The Turning Point," *New York Review of Books*, February 5, 1998.

91. Nick Thorpe, "Mladic Arrest Stirs Unhappy Memories in Sarajevo," BBC *News-Europe*, May 27, 2011. Food was so scarce that people not only ate grass but also dined on tree bark. See MacLean and Danziger, *Missing Lives*, 87.

92. Quoted in Mark Danner, "The U.S. and the Yugoslav Catastrophe."

93. Sudetic, *Blood and Vengeance*, 100.

94. Quoted in *Justice Report*, "Angelina Jolie Tackles the Issue of Wartime Rape," February 16, 2012, at www.birn.edu.com.

95. Quoted in *Justice Report*, "Wartime Rape."

96. *Justice Report*, "Wartime Rape."

97. E.M. quoted in *Justice Report*, "Vlahovic: Rape of Pregnant Woman," February 15, 2012, at www.birn.eu.com.

98. Toal and Dahlman, *Bosnia Remade*, 6.

99. Roger Cohen, "CIA Report on Bosnia Blames Serbs for 90% of War Crimes," *New York Times*, March 9, 1995.

100. "Srebrenica Genocide," July 9, 2007, 2, at www.srebrenicagenocide.org.

101. Quoted in "Srebrenica Genocide," July 9, 2007, 10, at www.srebrenicagenocide.org.

102. Mark Danner, "Bosnia: Breaking the Machine," *New York Review of Books*, February 19, 1998.

103. Quoted in Roy Gutman, "Dutch Reveal Horrors of Mission Impossible," *Newsday*, July 24, 1995.

104. Quoted in Daria Sito-Sucic and Maja Zuvela, "Srebrenica Recalled with Grief and Shame," *Washington Post*, July 12, 2005, A14.

105. See Citizen Association: Women of Srebrenica, March 1, 2004, 1, at http://srebrenica.net/index.en.php?link=uvod.

106. Lauren Comiteau, "Court Says the Dutch Are to Blame for Srebrenica Deaths," *Time*, July 6, 2011.

107. Quoted in Comiteau, "Court Says the Dutch Are to Blame."

108. "The Netherlands Liable for Deportation of More than Three Hundred Men in Srebrenica," *De Rechtspraak*, The Hague, July 16, 2014, at www.rechtspraak.nl.

109. Holbrooke, *To End a War*, 69. The ICTY, established in 1993, called the Srebrenica tragedy "the single worst atrocity committed in Yugoslavia during the wars of the 1990s." Afterward, nearly two dozen Serb leaders, from Generals Mladic, Krstic, and Radovan Karadzic to lower echelon military officers, were charged with committing war crimes and genocide. In its judgments indicting the leaders of the Srebrenica horrors, the ICTY concluded that many Serb actions constituted "genocide."

110. According to ICRC data, in 2005 there were 8,105 victims; in 2006, the number increased to 8,372; in 2007, there were 8,460 victims identified. Of that number, 78 percent were civilian dead (including 441 children) and 22 percent military dead. International Criminal Tribunal for the Former Yugoslavia (ICTY), "Outreach" Document, at www.icty.org/index-b.html.

111. Quoted in Mark Danner, "Bosnia: The Great Betrayal," *New York Review of Books*, March 26, 1998 (transcript of Serb radio communications).

112. Quoted in Roy Gutman, "The UN's Deadly Deal: How Troop-hostage Talks Led to Slaughter of Srebrenica," *Newsday*, May 29, 1996 (transcript of Serb radio communications).

113. *Gendercide Watch: The Srebrenica Massacre*, at www.gendercide.org /case_srebrenica.html. See also David Rohde, *Endgame*, 351, 353.

114. See studies published by *Association of Rape Victims in Sarajevo, Zene-Zrtve Rata (Women-Victims of War)*, www.srebrenicagenocide .org. A part of the solution to the Muslim "problem" was "rape warfare." A document issued by the Serb military outlined this strategy for eliminating the Muslims from the Greater Serbia: "Our analysis of the behavior of Muslim communities demonstrates that the morale, will, and bellicose nature of these groups can be undermined only if we aim our action at the point where the religious and social structure is most fragile. We refer to the women, especially adolescents, and to the children. Decisive intervention (rape) on these social figures would spread confusion, this causing first of all fear and then panic, leading to a possible retreat from the territories involved in war activity." See Allen, *Rape Warfare*.

115. Quoted in "Srebrenica Genocide," July 9, 2007, 13, at www.srebrenica genocide.org.

116. Mark Danner, "The Killing Fields of Bosnia," *New York Review of Books*, September 24, 1998, at www.gendercide.org.

117. This was, through 2014, the maximum penalty imposed by the ICTY. See "Srebrenica Killers Jailed for 553 Years So Far," *Balkan Transitional Justice*, July 11, 2013, at www.balkaninsight.com.

118. Quotes from "Srebrenica Genocide," July 9, 2007, 7, at www .srebrenicagenocide.org. In July 2013 Judge Meron, the president of the ICTY, quoting from the Karadzic trial proceedings, acknowledged that evidence presented clearly showed that "in meetings with Karadzic, 'it had been decided that one-third of Muslims would be killed, one-third would be converted to the Orthodox religion and a third will leave [Bosnia] on their own' and thus all Muslims would disappear from Bosnia." Quoted in Marlise Simons, "Genocide Charge Reinstated Against Wartime Leader of the Serbs," *New York Times*, July 11, 2013.

119. International Criminal Tribunal for the Former Yugoslavia, "Outreach" Document, at www.icty.org/index-b.html. Colonel Beara was tried for genocide and convicted by the ICTY in 2010. He was sentenced to life imprisonment. See also *Amnesty International Annual Report 2011—Bosnia and Herzegovina*, May 13, 2011, at www.unhcr.org.

120. Quoted in "Srebrenica Killers Jailed for 553 Years So Far."

121. Quoted in "Srebrenica Killers Jailed for 553 Years So Far."

122. See "Srebrenica Killers Jailed for 553 Years So Far."

123. United States Ambassador to the UN Madeline Albright presented a number of the photographs taken by the American spy satellites. See Citizen Association: Women of Srebrenica, March 1, 2004, 2, at http://srebrenica.net/index.en.php?link=uvod.

124. International Criminal Tribunal for the Former Yugoslavia, "Outreach" Document, at www.icty.org/index-b.html. Documents presented to the ICTY indicate that chemical weapons were used by the Serbs against the Muslims as early as 1993.

125. The Dayton Peace Accords, signed November 30, 1995, ushered in a new phase in the history of the South Slavs. Chapter Five will examine the Accords and what has happened since 1995.

126. See, generally, Holbrooke, *To End A War*.

127. See, for example, Nick Hawton, "Bosnia's Largest Mass Grave," BBC News, July 30, 2003, at www.news.bbc.co.uk. And Almir Arnaut, "Srebrenica Remains Found in Largest Mass Grave," *Washington Post*, August 17, 2006, at www.washingtonpost.org.

128. AP, "Bosnia: Bones of War Victims Found," *New York Times*, August 11, 2010.

129. Marija Arnautovic, "Bosnia: U N Urges Progress on Disappeared," *Institute for War and Peace Reporting*, June 28, 2010, at www.iwpr.net/global-voices/bosnia-un-urges-progress-disappeared.

3. Finding, Exhuming, and Identifying Remains

Epigraphs: "Bones Arriving Too Late," *Dani*, Sarajevo, Bosnia, April 28, 2000, at www.cdsp.neu.edu. Cox et al., *Scientific Investigation of Mass Graves*, 57. I am greatly indebted to Margaret Cox and her colleagues for their seminal research on forensic work in war zones.

1. See chapter 5 for the major problems that continue to plague the post-1995 nation.

2. Cox et al., *Scientific Investigation of Mass Graves*, 109.

3. Cox et al., *Scientific Investigation of Mass Graves*, 111.

4. Henrik Pryser Libell, "Grave of the Blue Butterflies," at www.bosnia massgraves.com.

5. Danny Rinehart, "Excavations of Skeletal Remains from an Anthropological Point of View," at www.rinehartforensics.com.

6. Interview, Amor Masovic, Sarajevo, Bosnia, April 2003. One Croat survivor said, "I hope in time those individuals who have such information will finally speak out, because their conscience will make them do so." Quoted in Ajdin Kamber, "Thousands of Bosnians Still Missing," *Institute for War and Peace Reporting*, May 25, 2011, at www.iwpr.net.

7. Wagner, *To Know Where He Lies*, 98.

8. Amer Jahid, "News: An Insider Reveals a Mass Grave near Prijedor," *Justice Report*, September 6, 2013, at www.justice-report.com.

9. Quoted in Denis Dzidic, "Bosnia's Biggest Mass Grave Raises Justice Hopes," *Justice Report*, January 30, 2014, at www.justice-report.com.

10. Quoted in MacLean and Danziger, *Missing Lives*, 59.

11. Quoted in Kamber, "Thousands of Bosnians Still Missing."

12. Stover and Shigekane, "The Missing in the Aftermath of War," 853.

13. Ironically, the signing was announced the day before the annual U N-sponsored commemorative International Day of the Disappeared.

14. Quoted in Sanela Gakovic, "Ex-Yugoslav Presidents Sign Missing Persons Declaration," Balkan Transitional Justice, August 29, 2014, at www.balkaninsight.com. The U N's representative at the signing, Flavia Pansieri, called it a "historic day."

15. Quoted in Kamber, "Thousands of Bosnians Still Missing."

16. Clea Koff interview, N O W, P B S, July 9, 2004.

17. Koff, *The Bone Woman*, 208.

18. Quoted in Libell, "Grave of the Blue Butterflies." These actions have delayed the identification process. "In some cases," said Amor Masovic (MPI), "we've gathered the remains of one person from 10 different bags containing remains." Because of this dilemma, more than 3,000 exhumed remains have not been identified as of 2010. See Aida Alie and Merima Husejnovie, "Uncertainty Ends for Families of Some Missing Bosnians," *Justice Report*, at www.balkaninsight.com.

19. Sandy MacIntyre, "Mass Grave in Bosnian Çave," *Allegheny Times*, March 21, 1996, A1.

20. Wagner, *To Know Where He Lies*, 83–84. The tactic "destroys the physical integrity of human remains . . . by the comingling and separating of bodies to the point where they are indistinguishable as individual skeletal remains" (84).

21. Harry Kreisler, "Voices from the Graves: Conversations with William Haglund," *Conversations With History, Institute of International Studies UC Berkeley*, September 22, 2000, at www.globetrotter.berkeley.edu.

22. Koff, *The Bone Woman*, 194.

23. Clea Koff wrote: "the people who committed the crimes we would be uncovering were still at large." Koff, *The Bone Woman*, 140.

24. Stover and Peress, *The Graves*, 96.

25. In some parts of Bosnia, Russian military forces were deployed to maintain order and protection. In the vicinity of Vukovar, Croatia, the Russians guarded the gravesites at night. Stover and Peress, *The Graves*, 99.

26. Koff, *The Bone Woman*, 149.

27. Koff, *The Bone Woman*, 142–43.

28. Libell, "Grave of the Blue Butterflies."

29. Farbridge, "Grave Hunters."

30. Beth Kampschror, "New Forensic Techniques Aid Efforts to Find Bosnia's War-Crimes Victims," *Christian Science Monitor*, August 25, 2005.

31. Kampschror, "New Forensic Techniques."

32. ICMP, "ICMP Finds Improved Methods for Locating Mass Graves," September 16, 2005, at www.ic-mp.org.

33. ICMP, "ICMP Finds Improved Methods for Locating Mass Graves."

34. Eric Bland, "New Tech Sees Dead People," *Discovery News*, April 16, 2010, at www.discovery.org. "Plants that grow on human graves are altered by the soil mixture below."

35. "Remote sensing works on the premise that every object emits a signal based on the waves of the electromagnetic spectrum it reflects back from the sun." Farbridge, "Grave Hunters."

36. Bland, "New Tech Sees Dead People."

37. Sassoli and Touga, "The ICRC and the Missing," 744.

38. Elizabeth Neuffer, "Mass Graves," in *Crimes of War: A–Z Guide*, at www.crimesofwar.com.

39. ICMP, *Locating and Identifying Missing Persons: A Guide For Families in Bosnia and Herzegovina*, 2010, at www.ic-mp.org.

40. ICMP, *Locating and Identifying Missing Persons: A Guide For Families in Bosnia and Herzegovina*, 2010.

41. Cox et al., *Scientific Investigation of Mass Graves*, 76.

42. Cox et al., *Scientific Investigation of Mass Graves*, 79–80.

43. Rinehart, "Excavations of Skeletal Remains," at www.crime-scene -investigator.net.

44. Quoted in Matthew Brunwasser, "In Srebrenica, a Memorial Brings Peace," *New York Times*, May 30, 2011.

45. DNA, *deoxyribonucleic acid*, "is a microscopic chain-like molecule that makes up the hereditary material found in nearly all the cells of the human body. Half of DNA is inherited from the mother, the other half from the father. DNA contains the biological information that is used by nature to build and maintain a person's body, and determines many of the distinctive characteristics of an individual. Except for twins, no two people share the same DNA pattern." ICMP, "Locating and Identifying," at www.ic-mp.org. Rinehart, "Excavation of Skeletal Remains," at www.crime-scene-investigator.net.

46. "The Law establishes the principles for improving the tracing process, the definition of a missing person, the method of managing the central records, realization of social and other rights of family members of missing persons, and other issues related to tracing missing persons from/in Bosnia and Herzegovina." LAW ON MISSING PERSON, CHAPTER I—GENERAL PROVISIONS, Article 1, (Subject of the Law). Another Article (7) created the agency responsible for implementing the law, the Missing Persons Institute (MPI), in order to improve the process of tracing missing persons and expedite identifications of mortal remains of missing persons. At www.ic-mp.org.

Article 2, Section 7 states: "An identified missing person is a person for whom, during the process of identification, it has been reliably determined that the mortal remains correspond to the specific person's physical, hereditary, or biological characteristics, or if the missing person appears alive. The process of identification shall be conducted in accordance with the laws applicable in Bosnia and Herzegovina." At www.ic-mp.org.

47. Antemortem means "preceding death."

48. *Conversations with History*: Institute of International Studies, University of California, Berkeley, California, "Human Rights Work: Conversation with Eric Stover," February 16, 1999, at www.globetrotter .berkeley.edu/people/Stover/stover-con99-1.html. See also Stover and Peress, *The Graves*, 163–73.

49. Stover and Peress, *The Graves*, 173.

50. Koff, *The Bone Woman*, 138–39.

51. Koff, *The Bone Woman*, 178.

52. Rinehart, "Excavations of Skeletal Remains."

53. Alicia Stevenson and Jonathan Dotan, "Report from Sarajevo: Identifying the Missing," UCLA *International Institute*, May 29, 2003, at www.intl@international.ucla.edu.

54. Quoted in Stevenson and Dotan, "Report from Sarajevo."

55. Wagner, *To Know Where He Lies*, 101–2.

56. Brunwasser, "In Srebrenica."

57. Andrew Carter, "DNA Clues to Bosnia's Missing," BBC News, January 21, 2002, at www.bbcn.com.

58. ICMP, at www.ic-mp.org/icfact.asp. See Carter, "DNA Clues to Bosnia's Missing."

59. ICMP, "Locating and Identifying Missing Persons," 14, at www.ic -mp.org.

60. ICMP, "Locating and Identifying Missing Persons," 11–13, at www .ic-mp.org.

61. Quoted in Alic and Husejnovic, "Uncertainty Ends," at www.balkan insight.com.

62. Quoted in Alic and Husejnovic, "Uncertainty Ends," at www.balkan insight.com.

63. Wagner, *To Know Where He Lies*, 117.

64. Koff interview, NOW, PBS.

65. Koff interview, NOW, PBS.

66. Koff, *The Bone Woman*, 194, 196.

67. Wagner, *To Know Where He Lies*, 108–15. See also the ICMP guide prepared for the families of the missing, *Locating and Identifying Missing Persons: A Guide for Families in Bosnia and Herzegovina*, May 2011. See also Koff, *The Bone Woman*, 169.

68. See generally, ICMP: *Locating and Identifying Missing Persons: A Guide for Families in Bosnia and Herzegovina*, 2011, at www.ic-mp.org.

69. Wagner, *To Know Where He Lies*, 159.

70. UN Commission on Human Rights, "Question of Enforced or Involuntary Disappearances," January 15, 1997, 4, at www.hri.ca/fortherecord 1997/documentation.

71. UN Commission on Human Rights, "Question of Enforced or Involuntary Disappearances," 5–6.

72. UN Commission on Human Rights, "Question of Enforced or Involuntary Disappearances," 6, 9.

73. See Annie Brown, "Scots Forensic Expert Tells of Mass Grave Horror," *Daily Record*, May 28, 2011, at www.dailyrecord.co.uk, and Christian Jennings, "Gunning for the Butchers of Bosnia," *Daily Mail*, February 9, 2007, at www.dailymail.co.uk.

74. See Columbian College of A&S, George Washington University, "For War Victims GW Alumnus Finds Missing Pieces of the Puzzle," September 2009, at www.columbian.gwu.edu.

75. The Geneva Convention of 1864 was the work of the founder of the ICRC, Henri Dunant. The modern guidelines were promulgated in the four Geneva Conventions of 1949 and the Additional Protocols of 1977.

76. ICRC, "Founding and Early Years of the ICRC," May 12, 2010, at www.icrc.org.

77. ICRC, *The ICRC: Its Mission and Work*, 2010, at www.icrc.org.

78. ICRC, *The ICRC: Its Mission and Work*, 2010, at www.icrc.org.

79. ICRC, *Missing Persons and International Humanitarian Law*, October 20, 2010, at www.icrc.org.

80. ICRC, *The ICRC in the Western Balkans*, October 29, 2010, at www.icrc.org.

81. ICRC, "Bosnia and Herzegovina," May 26, 2010, at www.icrc.org /web/doc.

82. Sassoli and Touga, "The ICRC and the Missing."

83. Sassoli and Touga, "The ICRC and the Missing," 728.

84. Stover and Shigekane, "The Missing in the Aftermath of War," 855.

85. ICRC, *Report: Families of Missing Persons: Responding to Their Needs*, August 2009, 4, at www.icrc.org. See also Stover and Shigekane, "The Missing in the Aftermath of War," 855.

86. Stover and Peress, *The Graves*, 196.

87. Sassoli and Touga, "The ICRC and the Missing," 728.

88. ICMP, "About ICMP," November 2008, at www.ic-mp.org.

89. See Christian Jennings, "Finding the Bodies to Fill the Bosnian Graves," *Scotsman*, September 12, 2007, at www.newscotsman.com.

90. Quoted in speech by Kathryne Bomberger, ICMP Director-General, at the International Association of Genocide Scholars, July 9–13, 2007, at www.ic-mp.org.

91. Press conference at the U.S. Department of State, Washington DC, November 7, 1997, at www.state.gov. Two years later, the Director-

General of the ICMP, Kathryne Bomberger, complained about the lack of cooperation between the entities: "I would like to express disappointment on a central issue relating to missing persons—the reluctance of Bosnian authorities to provide information on the fate of 'detainees unaccounted for.' It is also our hope that Croatia and Serbia can learn to cooperate with each other and recognize that mutual distrust . . . is a dead end." Speech, March 26, 1999, at www.ic-my.org.

92. Eldin Hadžović, "Sarajevo Shuns Recognition of Bosniak War Crimes," *Balkan Insight*, December 23, 2011, at www.balkaninsight.com. "Sixteen years after the Dayton Accord, which ended the war in Bosnia, Sarajevo authorities show little willingness to tackle crimes committed against Serb and Croatian civilians by the mainly Bosniak [Muslim] Army of Bosnia and Herzegovina during the siege."

93. ICMP, *Southeast Europe* (November 2008), at www.ic-mp.org.

94. High-throughput screening is a method for scientific experimentation allowing a researcher to quickly conduct necessary chemical, genetic, or pharmacological tests. ICMP, "About ICMP" (November 2008), at www.ic-mp.org.

95. ICMP, "15 Years: ICMP Fact Sheet," at www.ic-mp.org.

96. Samira Krehic, Sarajevo Office of ICMP, in September 29, 2010 interview, One World See, at www.oneworldsee.org.

97. Jennings, "Finding the Bodies."

98. Department of Global Health and Social Medicine, "Carola Eisenberg Speaks on Physicians for Human Rights," Harvard University, January 9, 2009, at www.harvard.edu.

99. Included among the dozens of nations PHR teams worked in are "Brazil, Israel, Czechoslovakia, Guatemala, Honduras, El Salvador, Iraqi Kurdistan, Iraq, Kuwait, Mexico, Panama, Rwanda, Thailand, the former Yugoslavia and very recently, Afghanistan." Cordner and McKelvie, "Developing Standards," 868.

100. Levin, "Physicians for Human Rights," 537.

101. Levin, "Physicians for Human Rights," 537.

102. PHR, "How We Work," February 2011, at www.phr.org.

103. PHR, "Justice and Forensic Science," December 13, 2011, at www.phr.org.

104. PHR, "International Forensic Program Training Programs," December 2011, at www.phr.org.

105. In the Republika Srpska, it was the Office for Tracing Detained and Missing Persons; in the Federation, it was the Federation Commission for Missing Persons.

106. Kirsten Juhl, "Institute for Missing Persons Gives Hope for Peace in the Balkans," *Innovations Report*, November 28, 2008, at www.uis.no /frontpage/news/article12384–132.html.

107. Kathryne Bomberger, quoted in ICMP, *Bosnia and Herzegovina*, November 2008, at www.ic-mp.org. Dr. Kirsten Juhl commented on the importance of this landmark action: "When work is lifted from the [entities] to a common institute of state level, [they] have to work with each other. The creation of the MPI is therefore a huge gain for peace and societal stability." Juhl, "Institute for Missing Persons."

108. ICMP, Bosnia and Herzegovina, November 2008, at www.ic-mp .org.

109. Quoted in ICMP, "Council of Ministers Formally Approves Missing Persons Institute," August 5, 2005, at www.ic-mp.org.

4. Forensic Scientists at Work

Epigraph: Quoted in Stover and Peress, *The Graves*, 10.

1. Harry Kreisler, *Conversations with History: William Haglund*, PHR, "Voices From the Graves," University of California, Berkeley, Institute of International Studies, September 22, 2000, at www.globetrotter.berkeley .edu. Forensic means "legal" and relates to the use of science in the investigation and detection of crimes that may lead to legal proceedings against the perpetrators.

2. Cordner and McKelvie, "Developing Standards," 870.

3. Quoted in Kreisler, "Voices from the Graves: Conversations with William Haglund."

4. Koff interview, NOW, PBS.

5. Komar and Buikistra, *Forensic Anthropology*, 246.

6. Stover and Shigekane, "The Missing in the Aftermath of War," 858.

7. Stover and Shigekane, "The Missing in the Aftermath of War," 846. Blewitt said directly: "We just don't have the resources to identify every single victim," 858.

8. Stover and Shigekane, "The Missing in the Aftermath of War," 847.

9. Quoted in Kreisler, "Voices from the Graves: Conversations with William Haglund."

10. Quoted in Kreisler, "Voices from the Graves: Conversations with William Haglund."

11. Haglund, quoted in Stover and Shigekane, "The Missing in the Aftermath of War," 845.

12. Quoted in Queenie Wong, "Local Scientist Uncovered Mass Graves in Bosnia," *Seattle Times*, May 26, 2011. Haglund was contracted

by the ICTY's prosecutor's office to be the senior forensic consultant to help find, exhume, and gather physical evidence from the mortal remains of Bosniak dead.

13. Quoted in Kreisler, "Voices from the Graves: Conversations with William Haglund."

14. In Argentina, in the effort to find the disappeared after the country's seven-year "dirty war" ended, the families created two potent NGOs, the Mothers of the Plaza de Mayo and the Grandmothers of the Plaza de Mayo. They conducted weekly protests demanding that the new leaders find their disappeared.

15. See BBC World News Service, "Dr. Clyde Snow," July 14, 2009, at www.bbc.co.uk.

16. Ferlini, *Silent Witness*, 169–70.

17. For example, Guatemala's military dictatorship, from 1962 through 1993, executed more than two hundred thousand Mayan Indians and buried the bodies in secret mass graves. After their rule ended, the insistent demand from survivors of the disappeared that the government find their missing led to the creation in 1997 of the Guatemala Forensic Anthropology Foundation (FAFG). This NGO, like all others, performs its work in Guatemala at the request of the Public Prosecutor's Office. Ferlini, *Silent Witness*, 174.

18. Komar and Buikistra, *Forensic Anthropology*, 21.

19. See generally Suzanne Bell, *The Facts on File Dictionary of Forensic Science*.

20. See generally Holbrooke, *To End A War*. Holbrooke, an American diplomat, was the major force that led to the signing of the Dayton Peace Accords, which ended the Bosnian wars in November 1995.

21. Bosnia consists of two entities: The Federation consists of a majority of Bosnian Croat and Muslim citizens. The other entity, populated by a majority of Bosnian Serbs, is the Republika Srpska.

22. Libell, "Grave of the Blue Butterflies."

23. Libell, "Grave of the Blue Butterflies."

24. The body was found in 2000, before the DNA process was implemented.

25. Interview with Nerzuk Curak, "Story from the Center of the Earth," *DANI*, August 2000.

26. Interview, March 2003, Sarajevo, Bosnia.

27. For example, see her stories, published in *The Magazine of the ICRC and Red Crescent Movement*, entitled "The Missing: A Hidden Tragedy," 2010, and "Summer [Camp] Break for 'Children of the Bosnia Missing,'" 2004.

28. Quoted in Laura Shin, "On the Job: Grave Testimony," *Stanford University Alumni Association Newsletter*, March–April 2005, at www.stanford.edu.

29. Shin, "On the Job."

30. Shin, "On the Job."

31. Interview with Judy Miller, "'Bone Woman' Digs Up Remains to Foil Killers," ABC *World News Tonight*, July 10, 2005, at www.abc.org.

32. Quoted in Jane Perlez, "A 'Bone Woman' Chronicles the World's Massacres," *New York Times*, April 24, 2004.

33. Koff, *The Bone Woman*, 160.

34. Koff, *Bone Woman*, 181.

35. Koff, *Bone Woman*, 180.

36. Koff, *The Bone Woman*, 275–76.

37. Kleck, "Working with Traumatised Women," 346.

38. "The word 'trauma' is of Greek origin and means wound. In a psychological context, it describes a 'wound to the soul.' People who have endured unimaginable brutality, who have faced death or have been forced to witness the torture and death of others often find it impossible to cope with everyday life afterwards and suffer a range of clinical symptoms." Kleck, "Working with Traumatised Women," 344–45. Regarding an injury inflicted by a familiar person, recall the heinous comment of the Croatian civilian to his neighbor, an ethnic Serb, in 1991: "You never expected us to be the ones to kill you. We are happy to surprise you."

39. Quoted in Mike O'Connor, "Muslim Women in Bosnia Try to Rebuild Lives without Men," *New York Times*, July 13, 1996, at www.nytimes.com.

40. Pasagic, "Psychosocial Recovery," 46.

41. O'Connor, "Muslim Women in Bosnia."

42. Pasagic, "Psychosocial Recovery," 47, 48.

43. Dr. Pasagic, quoted in Associated Press, "Work to Save Traumatized Generation Begins," USA *Today*, February 14, 1996, at www.usatoday.org.

44. Dr. Pasagic, "Work to Save Traumatized Generation Begins."

45. 2005 Alexander Langer Award Presentation, "Irfanka Pasagic: Carrier of Hope," at www.osservatoriobalcani.org.

46. Bosnia and Herzegovina-Projects, at www.info@projectsforpeace.org. See also Adopt Srebrenica, 2004–2012, at www.alexanderlanger.org.

47. Dybdahl and Pasagic, "Traumatic Experiences and Psychological Reactions Among Women in Bosnia During the War."

48. Pasagic, "Psychosocial Recovery in Bosnia," 49.

49. In this case, the ICJ ruled that genocide occurred in Srebrenica but that Serbia was not directly engaged in the action, and therefore the 1949 Convention on the Prevention and Punishment of Genocide did not apply. The ICJ concluded, however, "that Serbia violated its obligation under the Genocide Convention to prevent genocide in Srebrenica and by failing fully to cooperate with the ICTY." See Press Release 2007/8, 91 ICJ February 26, 2007. See also Courtney Angela Brkic's comments regarding the politics surrounding the ICJ decision and the "disbelief" the opinion engendered. Brkic, "Justice Denied in Bosnia," *Dissent* (Summer 2007), at www.dissentmagazine.org/article.

50. Report of Proceedings, "Reparations for Victims of Genocide, Crimes Against Humanity, and War Crimes: Systems in Place and Systems in the Making," *Redress, Seeking Reparation for Torture Victims*, at www.redress.org.

51. Stover, interviewed by Harry Kreisler, *Interview with Eric Stover: Conversations with History*, at www.globetrotter.berkeley.edu/people/Stover/stover-con99-0.html.

52. Stover, interviewed by Harry Kreisler, 1999.

53. To date, Pierre Omidyar, the founder of eBay, and wife Pam have committed more than $1 billion to hundreds of human rights causes through individual gifts and four organizations they created—Omidyar Network, Humanity United, HopeLab, and the Ulupono (Hawaiian for "doing the right thing") Initiative.

54. Quoted in FRONTLINE/WORLD: Bosnia. *The Men Who Got Away—Investigating Mass Murder*, 2006, at www.pbs.org/frontline world/stories/bosnia502.

55. Barry Bergman, "The Human Rights Center at 15," *The Berkeleyan*, September 10, 2009.

56. Bergman, "Human Rights Center."

57. Kreisler, *Interview with Eric Stover.*

58. Stover, *The Witnesses*, 44.

59. Kreisler, *Interview with Eric Stover.*

60. FRONTLINE/WORLD, *Bosnia.*

61. Kreisler, *Interview with Eric Stover.*

62. Kreisler, *Interview with Eric Stover.*

63. Rachel Nuwer, "Reading Bones to Identify Genocide Victims," *At War: Notes From the Front Lines*, November 18, 2011, at www.atwar.blogs.nytimes.com.

64. Stover, quoted in Bergman, "Human Rights Center."

65. Stover, quoted in Bergman, "Human Rights Center."

66. Kreisler, *Interview with Eric Stover.*

67. Kreisler, *Interview with Eric Stover.*

68. "Scientists are human. It's sometimes very difficult to do this work," said Stover, in Nuwer, "Reading Bones."

69. Stover, quoted in Bergman, "Human Rights Center."

70. Stover, quoted in FRONTLINE/WORLD, *Bosnia.*

71. Stover, quoted in Bergman, "Human Rights Center."

72. Quoted in Esa Lilja, "At 60, Helena Ranta is Still Likely to Take off to a Trouble Spot at Short Notice," *Helsingin Sanomat,* June 7, 2005, at www.helsinginsanomat.fi.

73. Quoted in "The Dead Have Rights Too," *Helsinki University Bulletin, The Hub,* at www.helsinki.fi/hub/articles/?article=25.

74. Lilja, "At 60, Helena Ranta." Her forensic work at mass gravesites led to her having to "face drawn guns, car bombs, and spurious arrests, and once she was even used as a human shield." "The Dead Have Rights Too."

75. Quoted in Lilja, "At 60, Helena Ranta."

76. This was done to prevent the mortal remains—the physical evidence that would show "crimes against humanity"—from "disappearing" after forensic workers left work in the evening.

77. "The Dead Have Rights Too."

78. Quoted in "The Dead Have Rights Too."

79. This account of the Racak incident is based on news reports published in *Helsingin Sanomat* between 1999 and 2003. See www.helsinginsanotmat.fi.

80. *Helsingin Sanomat,* "Helena Ranta Testifies at Milosevic Trial in The Hague," March 13, 2003, at www.helsinginsanomat.fi.

81. Destro, "Finnish Investigator Helena Ranta to Testify at Milosevic Trial," *Helsingin Sanomat,* November 26, 2002, at www.helsinki-hs.net.

82. Destro, "Finnish Investigator Helena Ranta."

83. Quoted "The Dead Have Rights Too."

84. Quoted in "The Dead Have Rights Too."

85. Quoted in "The Dead Have Rights Too."

86. Brkic, quoted in Robert Birnbaum, "Interview: Courtney Angela Brkic," May 24, 2005, at www.identitytheory.com/interviews/birnbaum159.php.

87. Brkic, *The Stone Fields,* 19.

88. Quoted in editorial, "20th Century Horrors, Exhumed," *Los Angeles Times,* August 15, 2004, at www.latimes.com.

89. "Devastation, Self-Discovery in the Balkans," *Boston Globe*, August 22, 2004, at www.boston.com.

90. Courtney Angela Brkic, "Justice Denied in Bosnia," *Dissent* (Summer 2007), at www.dissentmagazine.org/article. See also BBC News, "Eyewitness: Unearthing Bosnia's Dead," February 11, 2002, at www.bbc.co.uk.

91. Brkic, *Stone Fields*, 93–94.

92. Brkic, *Stone Fields*, 95, 127–28.

93. Brkic, *Stone Fields*, 22–23. The survivors inspected the stitching and "would turn the photographs this way and that, struggling to remember the details of shirts and belts" (209–10).

94. Brkic, quoted in "Interview with Courtney Angela Brkic."

95. BBC News, "Eyewitness: Unearthing Bosnia's Dead," March 1, 2004, at www.bbc.co.uk.

96. *Stillness* was published by Farrar, Straus, and Giroux, in New York, 2003.

97. BBC News, "Eyewitness: Unearthing Bosnia's Dead," March 1, 2004.

98. Quoted in Kreisler, "Voices from the Graves: Conversations with William Haglund." The first exhumations for both the ICTY and the ICTR were done in 1996.

99. Quoted in Stover and Peress, *The Graves*, 209.

100. Koff, *Bone Woman*, 274.

101. Quoted in Shin, "On the Job."

102. Quoted in Kreisler, "Voices from the Graves: Conversations with William Haglund."

5. Stark Realities

Epigraph: Quoted in Andrew Carter, "DNA Clues to Bosnia's Missing," BBC News, January 21, 2002, at www.bbc.co.uk. Quoted in Tochman, *Like Eating a Stone*. Bosnian-Croat citizen quoted in Barbara Matejcic, "Vukovar Still Imprisoned by its Bloody Past," *Balkan Insight*, February 21, 2012, at www.balkaninsight.com.

1. Alison Smale, "Roots of Bosnian Protests Lie in Peace Accords of 1995," *New York Times*, February 15, 2014, A4.

2. The Serb president, Slobodan Milosevic, represented the absent Bosnian-Serb political leader, Radovan Karadzic.

3. Edward P. Joseph, "Bosnia's Day of Reckoning Demands Bold Action," *Balkan Insight*, February 7, 2014, at www.balkaninsight.com.

4. Julie Mertus, "False Dawn: Bosnia Ten Years after Dayton," *Foreign Policy in Focus*, November 23, 2005, at www.fpif.org.

5. Mirjana Kosic, "Bosnia and Herzegovina Today—The View From Tuzla," *Insight on Conflict*, May 18, 2011, at www.ioc.org.

6. Director Clapper, appointed in 2010, heads the U.S. national security intelligence community and is the principal advisor to the president in this critical area of foreign policy.

7. Clapper, quoted in Jakov M. Sinisa, "U.S. Intelligence Deems Macedonia, Bosnia, 'Volatile,'" *Balkan Insight*, January 31, 2014, at www.balkaninsight.com.

8. In February 2012 the ICMP, the ICRC, and the MPI produced a complete list of the disappeared in the 1992–1995 Bosnian war. There were thirty-five thousand missing but, in 2012, twenty-three thousand had been found, with roughly twelve thousand still missing. This new information, said Amor Masovic, would facilitate the search for those still missing as well as helping families of the missing access welfare benefits. Quoted in Zdravko Ljubas, "Bosnia Unveils Complete List of Missing Persons," *Balkan Transitional Justice*, February 4, 2012, at www.balkaninsight.com.

9. Joseph, "Bosnia's Day of Reckoning."

10. Quotation in subhead is attributed to an unidentified Bosnian-Serb, quoted in Tochman, *Like Eating a Stone*.

11. Smale, "Roots of Bosnian Protests."

12. Some critics maintain that there are 180 "ministers," 600 legislators, and more than 70,000 bureaucrats working in all political units in Bosnia in 2014 and that they receive about 50 percent of the state budget annually. For salaries see Aleksandar Hemon and Jasmin Mujanovic, "Stray Dogs and Stateless Babies," *New York Times*, February 21, 2014, at www.nytimes.com/2014/02/22/opinion/sunday. Also see Wolfgang Petritsch, "Bosnians are Hungry in Three Languages," *Balkan Insight*, February 19, 2014, at www.balkaninsight.com.

13. Matthew Parish, "Serb Machiavelli Has Bosnia's Future in His Hands," *Balkan Insight*, September 20, 2011, at www.balkaninsight.com.

14. Steven Erlander, "The Dayton Accords: A Status Report," *New York Times*, June 10, 1996.

15. Kornblum, quoted in Smale, "Roots of Bosnian Protests."

16. Kornblum, quoted in Smale, "Roots of Bosnian Protests."

17. See generally *Dayton Peace Accords on Bosnia*, Washington DC, U.S. State Department, March 30, 1996, at www.state.gov.

18. Erlander, "The Dayton Accords."

19. Summary of the Dayton Peace Agreement on Bosnia-Herzegovina, Fact Sheet Released by the Office of the Spokesman, November 30, 1995, at www.uminnesota.edu.

20. Erlander, "The Dayton Accords."

21. Quoted in "On This Day," December 14, BBC News, December 14, 2006, at www.bbc.co.uk.org.

22. Quoted in Elvira M. Jukic, "Bosnian Serbs Mark Anniversary Amid War Allegations," *Balkan Traditional Justice*, June 14, 2014, at www.balkaninsight.com. In November 2013 Dodik said that independence for RS will "one day fall like a pear in our hands just as, say, Scotland or Catalonia will also do." Quoted in Elvira M. Jukic, "Catalans Spurn Links with Bosnian Serbs," *Balkan Insight*, January 30, 2014, at www.balkaninsight.com.

23. Parish said that there exists "a ruthless logic of Bosnia politics." Parish, "Serb Machiavelli."

24. Conversations with History: Interview with Eric Stover, February 16, 1999, at www.globetrotter.berkeley.edu. In 2011, a journalist ruefully wrote, "Most People in Bosnia believe that their interests will be protected only by leaders of their own ethnicity." Daniel McLaughlin, "A Land Divided," *Irish Times*, July 9, 2011.

25. Julie Mertus, "False Dawn: Bosnia Ten Years After Dayton," *Foreign Policy in Focus*, November 23, 2005, at www.ips-dc.org. See also Roger Cohen, "Enough of the Daytonians," *New York Times*, July 18, 2013.

26. Mertus, "False Dawn."

27. Mertus, "False Dawn."

28. Mertus, "False Dawn."

29. Mertus, "False Dawn."

30. Valentin Inzko, "Bosnia Marks 15 Years Since Dayton," *Balkan Insight*, November 22, 2010, at www.balkaninsight.com.

31. Elvira Jukic, "School Dispute Revives Bitter Memories in Eastern Bosnia," *Balkan Insight*, October 25, 2013, at www.balkaninsight.com.

32. Quoted in Jukic, "School Dispute."

33. Elvira Jukic, "Bosnia Serbs to Scrap Deal on National Subjects," *Balkan Insight*, November 19, 2013, at www.balkaninsight.com. Undeterred, the Bosniak parents and their counsel filed a legal petition with the European Court of Human Rights, located in Strasbourg, France. Elvira Jukic, "Bosnia School Bias Protesters Mull Strasbourg Appeal," *Balkan Insight*, November 11, 2013, at www.balkaninsight.com.

34. Vlado Azinovic, "Editorial: The Allure of Analogy," *Democracy and Security in Southeastern Europe: Managing Crisis*, May 2011, at www.balkaninsight.com.

35. Steven Woehrel, "Bosnia: Current Issues and U.S. Policy," CRS *Report for Congress*, June 20, 2011. See also Parish, "Serb Machiavelli."

36. *Amnesty International Annual Report 2011—Bosnia and Herzegovina*, May 13, 2011, at www.unhcr.org/refworld.

37. International Crisis Group (ICG), "Federation of Bosnia and Herzegovina—A Parallel Crisis," *Relief Web Europe Report No. 209*, September 28, 2010, at www.reliefweb.int/node/369534. See also Sabina Arslanagic, "Bosnian Croat Federation 'Ungovernable,' says ICG," *Balkan Insight*, September 20, 2010, at www.balkaninsight.com.

38. *Amnesty International Annual Report.*

39. *Amnesty International Annual Report.*

40. Matejcic, "Croats Hold Roma and Muslims at Arm's Length."

41. *Amnesty International Annual Report.*

42. The AI report noted, "There is a backlog of up to 10,000 untried war crimes cases." A state policy to address this dilemma, adopted in 2008, has not been implemented.

43. Dzana Brkanic, "New Srebrenica Genocide Indictment," *Justice Report*, September 6, 2013, at www.justice-report.com. (The former Bosnian Serb soldier had been hiding in Israel for years.) Mirna Buljugic, "Sarajevo Police Chief (Bosnian Serb) Jailed for War Crimes," *Justice Report*, August 28, 2013, at www.justice-report.com.

44. *Amnesty International Annual Report.*

45. Quoted in "Bosnia's December Surprise," *The Economist: Eastern Approaches*, December 30, 2011, at www.economist.uk.com.

46. Elvira Jukic, "Inzko Laments Bosnia's Stagnation in UN Report," *Balkan Insight*, November 13, 2013, at www.balkaninsight.com. See also Elvira Jukic, "Bosnian Serb Chief Says Country Should Split," *Balkan Insight*, November 20, 2013, at www.balkaninsight.com.

47. Jukic, "Inzko Laments Bosnia's Stagnation in UN Report."

48. Stover interview.

49. Dan Bilefsky, "Protests Over Government and Economy Roil Bosnia," *New York Times*, February 7, 2014, A7.

50. Alison Smale, "Furious Bosnians Shut Down Central Sarajevo," *New York Times*, February 10, 2014, A8.

51. Barbara Matejcic, "Croats Hold Roma and Muslims at Arm's Length," *Balkan Insight*, November 11, 2011, at www.balkaninsight.com.

52. British Foreign Secretary William Hague's response to the continuing unrest and demonstrations in Bosnia, quoted in Smale, "Furious Bosnians Shut Down Central Sarajevo."

53. Bilefsky, "Protests Over Government and Economy Roil Bosnia."

54. Smale, "Roots of Bosnian Protests."

55. Smale, "Roots of Bosnian Protests."

56. Smale, "Furious Bosnians Shut Down Central Sarajevo."

57. Nidzara Ahmetasevic, "I and My Fellow 'Hooligans' Can't Stop Now," *Balkan Insight*, February 11, 2014, at www.balkaninsight.com.

58. Ahmetasevic, "I and My Fellow 'Hooligans.'"

59. Srecko Latal, an analyst for a research organization based in Sarajevo, quoted in Bilefsky, "Protests Over Government and Economy Roil Bosnia."

60. Marija Ristic, "Serbia, Croatia Meet Bosnian Leaders to 'Calm' Unrest," *Balkan Insight*, February 10, 2014, at www.balkaninsight.com.

61. Elvira M. Jukic, "Bosnia Protesters Press Demand for PM To Go," *Bosnia Insight*, February 11, 2014, at www.bosniainsight.com.

62. Smale, "Furious Bosnians Shut Down Central Sarajevo."

63. Florien Bieber, "Is Change Coming (Finally)? Thoughts on the Bosnian Protests," *Balkan Insight*, February 10, 2014, at www.balkan insight.com.

64. "Bosnia's December Surprise," *The Economist*.

65. The wording on the Visegrad monument before the change: "To all killed and missing Bosniak men, women, and child victims *of genocide* in Visegrad." After the excision of "of genocide"—but without the addition of "of crimes against humanity"—the wording became: "To all killed and missing Bosniak men, women, and child victims in Visegrad." See Denis Dzidic, "Bosnian Serbs Delete 'Genocide' From Visegrad Memorial," *Balkan Transitional Justice*, January 23, 2014, at www.balkaninsight.com.

66. Eldin Hadžović, "Sarajevo Shuns Recognition of Bosniak War Crimes," *Balkan Insight*, December 23, 2011, at www.balkaninsight.com.

67. WGEID Press Release of June 21, 2010, on the Visit to Bosnia, at www2.ohchr.org/english/issues/disappear/group/docs/PR 21.06.10.pdf.

68. More than 92 percent of the missing were Bosniaks. See Ljubas, "Bosnia Unveils Complete List."

69. Some of these groups are Association of Relatives of Missing Persons of the Sarajevo-Romanija Region, Association of Families of Killed and Missing Defenders of the Homeland, Association of Women—Victims of War, and Vive Zene Tuzla.

70. See generally *Written Information for the Examination of Bosnia and Herzegovina's Combined Second to Fifth Periodic Reports*, October 12, 2010, Swiss Association Against Impunity, at www.trial-ch.org; *Written Information for the Adoption of the List of Issues by the Human Rights Committee with Regards to Bosnia and Herzegovina's Second Periodic Report*, December 2011, at www.trial-ch.org; and UN General Assem-

bly, Human Rights Council, Sixteenth Session, Agenda Item 3, *Report of the* WGEID, *Mission to Bosnia and Herzegovina*, December 28, 2010. Quotes in the next section come from these reports.

71. The official mission of this organization, last posted in 2010, is "Operational Team of the Republic Srpska for Tracing Missing Persons." Formed in June 2008, its website is www.nestalirs.com/onama.html. In 2015 it remains in RS, merged into the RS Center for Researching War Crimes and Searching for Missing Persons. ICMP, *Bosnia and Herzegovina, Missing Persons from Armed Conflicts of the 1990s.* www.ic-mp.org.

72. CIA, DIA, NSC, SECD, SECS cables found in www.wikileaks.org/plusd/08SARAJEVO1531 _a.html.

73. Tanja Topic, quoted in Maja Bjelajac, "War of Words Over Missing Bosnian Serbs," *AlertNet (Reuters)*, February 18, 2011, at www.trust.org.

74. Bjelajac, "War of Words."

75. WGEID Report.

76. WGEID Report.

77. Amer Jahic, "An Insider Reveals a Mass Grave near Prijedor," *Justice Report*, September 6, 2013, at www.justice-report.com.

78. Associated Press, "Bosnia Digging Up What Could Be Biggest Mass Grave," *Burlington Free Press*, November 1, 2013, 3A.

79. Press release, "Countries of the Former Yugoslavia Need to Step Up Their Efforts to Resolve Cases of Missing Persons," Office of Commissioner for Human Rights, December 14, 2010, at www.commissioner.coe.int.

80. Azinovic, "Allure of Analogy."

81. Azinovic, "Allure of Analogy."

82. Marija Tausan, "EU Allocates 15[.8] Million for New Judges and Prosecutors," *Justice Report*, January 30, 2014, at www.justice-report.com.

83. Tausan, "EU Allocates 15[.8] Million."

84. From UN Human Rights Council, WGEID Report, "Mission to Bosnia," December 28, 2010, 16–19.

85. Boris Pavelic, "NGOs: War Crimes Victims in Croatia 'Forgotten,'" *Balkan Transitional Justice*, February 23, 2012, at www.balkaninsight.com.

86. See Selma Ucanbarlic, "Eyewitnesses to Oborci Killings Fade Away," *Balkan Investigative Reporting Network*, March 2, 2012, at www.birn.eu.com. The author writes about Bosniak and Croat massacres in a small town in 1992 and 1995 where the authorities have done nothing to bring the killers to justice. "As eyewitnesses to the killings age and in some cases die, fears are growing in the village soon

no one will remain to testify about the murders that have scarred their community."

87. Hawton, "Conflicting Truths."

88. Hawton, "Conflicting Truths."

89. Matthew Brunwasser, "In Srebrenica, a Memorial Brings Peace," *New York Times*, May 30, 2011.

90. Brunwasser, "In Srebrenica."

91. Quoted in McLaughlin, "A Land Divided."

92. Miodrag Stojanovic, "Verdicts Haven't Brought Reconciliation," *Balkan Insight*, February 14, 2012, at www.balkaninsight.com.

93. Quoted in Hadžović, "Sarajevo Shuns Recognition of Bosniak War Crimes."

94. AP, "Bosnia: Convicted War Criminal Welcomed as a Hero," *New York Times*, August 30, 2013, at www.nytimes.com/2013.

95. News report, "Bosnia Entities Argue Over Sochi Winter Games," *Balkan Insight*, January 30, 2014, at www.balkaninsight.com.

96. Edward P. Joseph, "Only Outside Intervention Can Break Bosnia's Deadlock," *Balkan Insight*, February 12, 2014, at www.balkan insight.com.

97. Quoted in Smale, "Roots of Bosnian Protests."

98. Cohen, "Enough of the Daytonians."

99. Refik Hodzic, International Center for Transitional Justice, quoted in Marija Tausan, "Karadzic Genocide Decision Divides Bosnians," *Justice Report*, July 11, 2013, at www.justice-report.com.

100. Agence France-Press, "Bosnian Serb Police Play down Shots Fired at Forensic Experts," July 28, 2010. See also *BBC Monitoring via COMTEX*, "MPI Investigators Shot At in Bosnian Serb Entity," July 28, 2010.

101. Denis Dzidic, "More Than 160 Victims Identified from Lake Perucac," *Balkan Transitional Justice*, February 13, 2012, at www.balkan insight.com.

102. ICMP, *Bosnia and Herzegovina, Missing Persons from Armed Conflicts of the 1990s: A Stocktaking*, 2014, at www.ic-mp.org.

BIBLIOGRAPHY

Allen, Beverly. *Rape Warfare: The Hidden Genocide in Bosnia and Croatia*. Minneapolis: University of Minnesota Press, 1997.

Ball, Howard. *Genocide*. Santa Barbara, CA: ABC-Clio, 2010.

———. *Prosecuting War Crimes and Genocide: The Twentieth Century Experience*. Lawrence: University Press of Kansas, 1999.

Blaauw, Margaret, and Virpi Lahteenmaki. "'Denial and Silence' or 'Acknowledgement and Disclosure.'" *International Review of the Red Cross* 84 (December 2003).

Bomberger, Kathryne. ICMP Director-General at the International Association of Genocide Scholars, July 9–13, 2007, at www.ic-mp.org.

Butolo, Willi, Maria Hagl, and Marion Kruesmann. *Life After Trauma: A Workbook for Healing*. New York: Guilford, 1999.

Cigar, Norman. *Genocide in Bosnia: The Policy of Ethnic Cleansing*. Lubbock: Texas A&M Press, 1997.

Clark, Christopher. *The Sleepwalkers: How Europe Went to War in 1914*. New York: Harper/Collins, 2013.

Cordner, Stephen, and Helen McKelvie. "Developing Standards in International Forensic Work to Identify Missing Persons." *International Review of the Red Cross* 84 (December 2002), 868.

Cox, Margaret, Ambika Flavel, Ian Hanson, Joanna Laver, and Roland Wessling. *The Scientific Investigation of Mass Graves: Towards Protocols and Standard Operating Procedures*. New York: Cambridge University Press, 2008.

Davidson, Basil. "Death of Josip Broz Tito." *History Today* 30, no. 10 (1980), at www.historytoday.com.

Dayton Peace Accords on Bosnia. Washington DC: U.S. State Department, March 30, 1996, at www.state.gov.

Dedijer, Vladimir. *The Yugoslav Auschwitz and the Vatican: The Croatian Massacre of the Serbs During World War Two.* Buffalo NY: Prometheus Books, 1992.

Dorfman, Ariel. *Widows.* New York: Penguin, 1983.

Dybdahl, Ragnhild, and Irfanka Pasagic. "Traumatic Experiences and Psychological Reactions Among Women in Bosnia During the War." *Medicine, Conflict and Survival* 16 (2000): 281–90.

Eisenberg, Carola. Department of Global Health and Social Medicine, "Carola Eisenberg Speaks on Physicians for Human Rights." Harvard University, January 9, 2009, at www.harvard.edu.

Farbridge, Peter. "Grave Hunters." *Headway: Research, Discover and Innovation at McGill University* 5, No. 2. (December 14, 2011).

Ferlini, Roxanna. *Silent Witness: How Forensic Anthropology Is Used to Solve the World's Toughest Crimes.* Ontario CA: Firefly Books, 2002.

Gutman, Roy. *A Witness to Genocide.* New York: Lisa Drew Books, 1993.

Hastings, Max. *Catastrophe 1914: Europe Goes to War.* New York: A. A. Knopf, 2013.

Hawton, Nick. "Conflicting Truths: The Bosnian War." *History Today* 59, no. 8 (2010), at www.historytoday.com.

Heleta, Savo. *Not My Turn To Die: Memoirs of a Broken Childhood in Bosnia.* New York: Amacom, 2008.

Herman, Judith. *Trauma and Recovery: The Aftermath of Violence—From Domestic Abuse to Political Terror.* New York: Basic Books, 1997.

Holbrooke, Richard C. *To End a War.* New York: Random House, 1998.

International Commission on Missing Persons. *Bosnia and Herzegovina, Missing Persons from Armed Conflicts of the 1990s: A Stocktaking.* 2014. www.ic-mp.org.

———*Locating and Identifying Missing Persons: A Guide For Families in Bosnia and Herzegovina.* 2010, at www.ic-mp.org.

International Committee of the Red Cross. Research and Documentation Center. *The Bosnian Book of the Dead.* June 21, 2007.

Kleck, Monika. "Working with Traumatised Women." In *Peacebuilding and Civil Society in Bosnia-Herzegovina: Ten Years After Dayton,* ed. Martina Fischer. Munster, Germany: Lit Verlag, 2006, at www.berghof-center.org.

Klemencic, Matjaz. "The Rise and Fall of Yugoslavia: From King Aleksandar to Marshall Tito, 1918–1980." In *The Slovenian,* 211–38, at www.slovenia.com.

Koff, Clea. *The Bone Woman: Among the Dead in Rwanda, Bosnia, Croatia, and Kosovo.* Sydney, Australia: Hodder Press, 2004.

Komar, Debra A., and Jane E. Buikistra. *Forensic Anthropology: Contemporary Theory and Practice.* New York: Oxford University Press, 2008.

Levin, Aaron. "Physicians for Human Rights." *Annals of Internal Medicine* 134, no. 6 (March 20, 2001), at www.annals.org.

Maass, Peter. *Love Thy Neighbor: A Story of War.* New York: Vintage, 1997.

MacLean, Rory, and Nick Danziger. *Missing Lives.* Stockport UK: Dewi Lewis Publishers, 2010.

Malcolm, Noel. *Bosnia: A Short History.* New York: NYU Press, 1996.

Mazower, Mark. *The Balkans: A Short History.* New York: Modern Library, 2002.

Pasagic, Irfanka. "Psychosocial Recovery in Bosnia in the Aftermath of Violence." In *Dealing with the Past in Post-Conflict Societies: Ten Years After the Peace Accords in Guatemala and Bosnia-Herzegovina,* ed. Jonathan Sisson. Swisspeace Foundation, January 2007.

Quirk, Gregory J., and Leonel Casco, "Stress Disorders of Families of the Disappeared." *Social Science and Medicine* 39, no. 12 (1994).

"Reparations for Victims of Genocide, Crimes Against Humanity, and War Crimes: Systems in Place and Systems in the Making." *Redress, Seeking Reparation for Torture Victims.* Peace Palace, The Hague, Netherlands, March 1–2, 2007, at www.redress.org.

Rinehart, Danny. "Excavations of Skeletal Remains from an Anthropological Point of View," at www.rinehartforensics.com.

Rohde, David. *Endgame: The Betrayal and Fall of Srebrenica, Europe's Worst Massacre Since World War II.* New York: Farrar, Straus, and Giroux, 1997.

Sassoli, Marco, and Marie-Louise Touga. "The ICRC and the Missing." *International Review of the Red Cross* 84, no. 848 (December 31, 2002), at www.icrc.org.

Serbian Academy of Arts and Sciences, "Serbian Academy of Arts and Sciences (SANU) Memorandum, 1986," at www.chnm.gmu.edu/1989/items/show/674.

Stover, Eric. *The Witnesses: War Crimes and the Promise of Justice in The Hague.* Philadelphia: University of Pennsylvania Press, 2005.

Stover, Eric, and Gilles Peress, *The Graves: Srebrenica and Vukovar.* Zurich, Switzerland: Scalo, 1998.

———, and Rachel Shigekane. "The Missing in the Aftermath of War: When Do the Needs of Victims' Families and International War Crimes Tribunals Clash?" *International Review of the Red Cross* 84 (December 2002).

Sudetic, Chuck. *Blood and Vengeance: One Family's Story of the War in Bosnia.* New York: Penguin, 1999.

Toal, Gerard, and Carl T. Dahlman. *Bosnia Remade: Ethnic Cleansing and Its Reversal.* New York: Oxford University Press, 2011.

Tochman, Wojciech. *Like Eating a Stone: Surviving the Past in Bosnia.* New York: Atlas and Co., 2011.

Wagner, Sarah E. *To Know Where He Lies: DNA Technology and the Search for Srebrenica's Missing.* Berkeley: University of California Press, 2008.

Woehrel, Steven. "Bosnia: Current Issues and U.S. Policy." CRS *Report for Congress.* Congressional Research Service, Washington DC, June 20, 2011.

Woodward, Susan L. *Balkan Tragedy: Chaos and Dissolution After the Cold War.* Washington DC: Brookings, 1997.

INDEX

prosecuting, 14–15, 89–90; rape as aspect of, 44; "safe havens" massacre as, 50; terminology, 143, 173n109, 190n65

geography, 64

geology, 95

Goldstone, Richard, 13, 87, 101

Government Commission for Detained and Missing Persons, 75

Grandmothers of the Plaza de Mayo, 92, 182n14

Group for Psychological Assistance to Traumatized Women and Camp Detainees, 106

Guatemala, 182n17

Guatemala Forensic Anthropology Foundation (FAFG), 182n17

Haglund, William, 181n12; in Cyprus, 161n24; on dangers of forensic science, 61; on exhaustion of excavation, 123; on humanitarian role of forensic science, 90–91

Halilovic, Sanela, 5

Hanson, Ian, 55

Hapsburg Empire, 25, 26, 165n21

Hastings, Max, 23, 165n18, 165n19, 166n26, 166n27

Hawton, Nick, 153

health care, 140

Heleta, Savo, 164n7

Herman, Judith, 9

High Judicial and Prosecutorial Council of Bosnia, 152

high-throughput screening, 82, 180n94

al-Hilla mass grave, 161n31

history of Balkans, 21–52; power of, 153–55

Hodzic, Ramiza, 125

Holbrooke, Richard, 49, 125, 128, 182n20

home, loss of, 7

hope: destroying, 79, 162n35; unreasonable, 7–8, 120

House of Friendship, 107

Huffine, Ed, 70

human remains: chemistry of, 64–65; identification of, 66–75, 89–92; moved and reburied, 53, 60–61, 64, 67, 176n18, 176n20; smuggled out of former Yugoslavia, 115, 185n76

Human Rights Council (HRC), 163n38

Human Rights Office Tuzla, 108

hyperspectral imaging, 64–65, 176n35

identification, 66–75; DNA method of, 69–71; high priority of, 90–92; low priority of, 89–90; organizations involved in, 75–86; protocol for, 72–74; slowness of traditional method of, 67–68

Identification Coordination Centers, 66. See also mortuaries

infant mortality, 140

information sharing, 85, 86

Institute for Missing Persons (IMP), 96. See also Missing Persons Institute (MPI)

Inter-Entity Boundary Line, 127

intermarriage, 22, 23

International Commission on Missing Persons (ICMP), 12, 79–82; Antemortem Database Project and, 81; co-founding Missing Persons Institute (MPI), 85; DNA tested by, 72, 80; expansion of, 91; formation of, 76; founding of, 79–80; legal aspect of work of, 82; mission of, 80

International Committee of the Red Cross (ICRC), 77–79, 98, 99–100; antemortem database and, 75, 98–99; Balkan Work Group, 98; and

Republika Srpska (RS), 127–28; Bosnian Spring and, 141–42; cooperating with Federation of Bosnia and Herzegovina, 85, 91, 96; creation of, 43, 171n87, 182n21; discriminating against Bosniak students, 134–35, 188n33; as part of Bosnia and Herzegovina, 52; possible secession of, 135, 136, 138, 188n22; withdrawal of, from MPI, 145–47. *See also* Bosnia and Herzegovina, Federation of

return, freedom of, 130–31

revenge, 10, 16

Rivzic, Adnan, 70

Rodrigues, Almiro, 50

Roma, 137

Rome Conference (1998), 15

Rwanda, 13, 14

"safe havens," xi; massacres in, 47–48, 49

Samira (guide), xiv

sappers, 63, 65

Sarajevo: Bosnian Spring and, 140, 141; as capital of Bosnia-Herzegovina, 130; siege of, 43–44, 172n91

satellite images, 63–64

school: ethnic controversy over, 133–35, 139, 188n33; as key to children's survival, 105–6; and trauma of teachers, 105

Serbian Academy of Arts and Sciences, 35

Serbian Democratic Party, 38

Serbian Empire, 22, 164n11

Serbian nationalism, 23–26, 34–38, 165n17, 166n26, 168n48; after Dayton Accords, 131, 138, 188n22; in epic songs, 24, 265n16; terrorist groups and, 24–26, 165n18

Serbian National Radical Party (NRS), 27

Serbs: in Bosnia, 38–39; at center of Balkan clashes, 21; chemical weapons used by, 174n124; denying genocide, 9, 60, 143, 156–57; ethnic cleansing strategy of, 41–42, 46, 173n114, 174n118; omitted from Croatian Constitution, 39; paramilitaries of, xi, xii, 43, 172n89; political obstruction by, 60, 135, 156–57; practicing ethnic cleansing, xii, 9, 40, 41–42, 46–47, 116–18, 159n3; radicalization of, 37; religion and, 22, 24; rewarded under Dayton Accords, 131–32; unification of, 36–38, 168n58; as victims of ethnic cleansing, 29–30, 41, 85, 146, 167n35, 167n37, 180n92

sewing as antemortem data, 69, 186n93

sifting earth, 66

silence, crime of, 59–60, 108, 155

Slavic ethnicity, 22–23, 164n7, 164n8, 166n27

Slavic states, medieval, 22

Slovenia, 34, 170n72

Snow, Clyde, 92, 93, 101, 112, 161n30; *Witnesses from the Grave*, 100

Sochi Winter Olympics (2014), 155

social media, 142

Solana, Javier, 48

Srebov, Vladimir, 42

Srebrenica, 112–13, 121–22, 184n49; denial of massacre in, 9, 136, 156–57, 161n27; glorification of murderers of, 136; memorial cemetery of, xiv, 154; physical evidence from, 69; siege of, 46–52, 173n109

Stepan Dusan (tsar), 164n11

Stillness (Brkic), 122

The Stone Fields (Brkic), 122

Stover, Eric, 92, 93, 109–14, 132; at Physicians for Human Rights (PHR), 110–11; on working in war zones, 110

Strinovic, David, 123
Sudetic, Chuck, 164n5, 170n74
Suljagic, Emir, xi–xii, 55
survivors: antemortem data provided by, 68, 69; blood reference samples of, 70, 71, 74; isolation of, 12; life stopping for, 6; of lost child, 5; material hardship for, 6–7, 104; needing closure, 74–75, 89–91, 113, 120; needing tangible body, 79; needing to hold funerals, 19; NGOs of, 91–92; number of, xvi; psychological support for, 104, 106–7, 137, 148; as refugees, 1; rights of, 151; Serbian violence against, xiii; suffering of, 4–10, 79, 113, 162n35; support of, 98, 99, 187n8; unable to mourn, 6, 7–8; victimized by being forgotten, 13. *See also* trauma

teeth. *See* odontology
Tenth Sabotage Battalion, 51
Tito (Josip Broz), 31–34, 167n42
Tomasica mine, 58–59
trauma, 183n38; and collective traumatization, 11, 103, 104–5; inflicted by a familiar person, 183n38
Treaty of Versailles, 165n24
Tripartite Pact, 29
truth, right to, 151
Tudjman, Franjo, 38, 39, 126, 169n67, 170n74
Tulic, Sajida, 139
Turks. *See* Ottoman Empire
Tuzla: Bosniak women and children sent to, 49, 104; Bosnian Spring and, 140, 141; mortuary at, 70
Tuzlanska Amica (NGO), 106, 107
Tuzla Orphanage, 107

Ucanbarlic, Selma, 191n86
unemployment, 139, 140, 141
Union or Death (Black Hand), 24

United Nations (UN): response of, to genocide, 14; "safe havens" unprotected by, 48
United Nations Commission on Experts, 61–62
United Nations High Commissioner for Refugees (UNHCR), 75
United Nations Protection Force (UNPROFOR), 48
Ustashe, 28, 38, 166n30, 167n33; in Argentina, 167n47; death squads, 29–30, 167n35; praise for, 39

Vance, Cyrus, 81
Vatican, 167n47
Vekic, Anisa Suceska, 1
village, destruction of, 104
violence, cycles of, 153, 154
Visegrad, 53, 157; vandalism of Bosniak memorial in, 143, 190n65
Vlahovic, Veselin "Batko," 45
Vollen, Laurie, 69
Vukovar hospital massacre, 40–41; investigation into, 41, 61–62, 87–88; Russian forces protecting gravesites, 176n25

"wages of denial," 9
Wagner, Sarah, 74
Walker, William, 116
war criminals: backlog in cases against, 189n42; bringing to justice, 2, 17, 44–45, 173n109; freedom of, 105, 121, 125, 137–38, 148, 153, 176n23; as heroes, 154, 155; names of, withheld from survivors, 2, 10; in positions of authority, xii, xv, 62; silence of, 148
wars, 160n5, 170n74, 170n75; aftermath of, 1; doing forensic science during, 110; increase of civilian casualties in, 14; number of victims of, 4, 142–43; in twentieth century, 14
Wessling, Roland, 55